ORTHOPEDIC CLINICS OF NORTH AMERICA

www.orthopedic.theclinics.com

Technological Advances

April 2023 • Volume 54 • Number 2

Editor-in-Chief
FREDERICK M. AZAR

ELSEVIER

1600 John F. Kennedy Boulevard • Suite 1800 • Philadelphia, Pennsylvania, 19103-2899.

http://www.orthopedic.theclinics.com

ORTHOPEDIC CLINICS OF NORTH AMERICA Volume 54, Number 2
April 2023 ISSN 0030-5898, ISBN-13: 978-0-323-93885-3

Editor: Megan Ashdown
Developmental Editor: Ann Gielou Posedio

Orthopedic Clinics of North America (ISSN 0030-5898) is published quarterly by Elsevier Inc., 360 Park Avenue South, New York, NY 10010-1710. Months of issue are January, April, July, and October. Business and Editorial Offices: 1600 John F. Kennedy Blvd., Suite 1800, Philadelphia, PA 19103-2899. Customer Service Office: 3251 Riverport Lane, Maryland Heights, MO 63043. Periodicals postage paid at New York, NY and additional mailing offices. Subscription prices are $365.00 per year for (US individuals), $834.00 per year for (US institutions), $433.00 per year (Canadian individuals), $1,019.00 per year (Canadian institutions), $501.00 per year (international individuals), $1,019.00 per year (international institutions), $100.00 per year (US students), $100.00 per year for (Canadian students), $220.00 per year for (international students). Foreign air speed delivery is included in all *Clinics* subscription prices. All prices are subject to change without notice. **POSTMASTER:** Send change of address to *Orthopedic Clinics of North America*, **Elsevier Health Sciences Division, Subscription Customer Service, 3251 Riverport Lane, Maryland Heights, MO 63043. Customer Service (orders, claims, online, change of address): Elsevier Health Sciences Division, Subscription Customer Service, 3251 Riverport Lane, Maryland Heights, MO 63043. Tel: 1-800-654-2452 (U.S. and Canada); 314-447-8871 (outside U.S. and Canada). Fax: 314-447-8029. E-mail:** journalscustomerservice-usa@elsevier.com **(for print support);** journalsonlinesupport-usa@elsevier.com **(for online support).**

Reprints. For copies of 100 or more, of articles in this publication, please contact the Commercial Reprints Department, Elsevier Inc., 360 Park Avenue South, New York, NY 10010-1710. Tel.: 212-633-3874; Fax: 212-633-3820; E-mail: reprints@elsevier.com.

Orthopedic Clinics of North America is covered in *MEDLINE/PubMed (Index Medicus)*, *Cinahl, Excerpta Medica, and Cumulative Index to Nursing and Allied Health Literature.*

EDITORIAL BOARD

CONTRIBUTORS

EDITOR

FREDERICK M. AZAR, MD
Professor, Department of Orthopaedic
Surgery and Biomedical Engineering, The
University of Tennessee Health Science
Center; Chief-of-Staff, Campbell Clinic,
Inc,Memphis, Tennessee, USA

AUTHORS

JAKOB ACKERMANN, MD
Orthopedic Resident, Department of
Orthopedics, Balgrist University Hospital,
University of Zurich, Zurich, Switzerland

KAZZANDRA ALANIZ, BS
Department of Bioengineering, Clemson
University, Clemson, South Carolina, USA; The
Clemson University Medical University of
South Carolina Bioengineering Program,
Charleston, South Carolina, USA

BRANDON ALLEN, BA
National Spine Health Foundation, Reston,
Virginia, USA

BRIELLE ANTONELLI, BA
Research Assistant, Department of
Orthopedic Surgery, Brigham and Women's
Hospital, Harvard Medical School, Boston,
Massachusetts, USA

MOHAMMAD T. AZAM, BS
Orthopaedic Surgery Research Fellow, Foot
and Ankle Division, Department of
Orthopaedic Surgery, NYU Langone Health,
New York, New York, USA

TYLER J. BROLIN, MD
Department of Orthopaedic Surgery and
Biomedical Engineering, The University of
Tennessee Health Science Center–Campbell
Clinic, Memphis, Tennessee, USA; Campbell
Clinic Orthopaedics, Germantown,
Tennessee, USA

JOSEPH E. BURKHARDT, DO
Bronson Orthopedic Specialists, Battle Creek,
Michigan, USA

JAMES J. BUTLER, MB, BCh
Orthopaedic Surgery Research Fellow, Foot
and Ankle Division, Department of
Orthopaedic Surgery, NYU Langone Health,
New York, New York, USA

ANTONIA F. CHEN, MD, MBA
Orthopedic Surgeon, Department of
Orthopedic Surgery, Brigham and Women's
Hospital, Harvard Medical School, Boston,
Massachusetts, USA

JAMES CHOW, MD
Chow Surgical LLC, Phoenix, Arizona, USA

JONATHAN R. DANOFF, MD
Attending Orthopedic Surgeon, Department
of Orthopedic Surgery, Northwell Health
Orthopedic Institute, Great Neck, New York,
USA

ZACHARY R. DILTZ, MD
Department of Orthopedic Surgery,
LeBonheur Children's Hospital, Department of
Orthopedic Surgery, The University of
Tennessee Health Science Center–Campbell
Clinic, Memphis, Tennessee, USA; Campbell
Clinic Orthopedics, Germantown, Tennessee,
USA

MATTHEW L. DUENES, MD
Orthopaedic Surgery Resident, Foot and
Ankle Division, Department of Orthopaedic
Surgery, NYU Langone Health, New York,
New York, USA

TRAVIS EASON, MD
Department of Orthopaedic Surgery and
Biomedical Engineering, The University of
Tennessee Health Science Center–Campbell
Clinic, Memphis, Tennessee, USA

MOHAN S.R. ELAPOLU, PhD
Department of Automotive Engineering, Clemson University, Greenville, South Carolina, USA

DAVID W. FABI, MD
San Diego Orthopaedic Associates Medical Group, Inc, San Diego, California, USA

ANDREAS FONTALIS, MD, MSc (Res), MRCS (Eng)
Department of Trauma and Orthopaedic Surgery, University College Hospital, Division of Surgery and Interventional Science, University College London, London, United Kingdom

ARIANNA L. GIANAKOS, DO
Foot and Ankle Surgery Fellow, Foot and Ankle Division, Department of Orthopaedic Surgery, NYU Langone Health, New York, New York, USA

DIA ELDEAN GIEBALY, MBChB, MSc, FRCS (Tr&Orth), eMBA
Department of Trauma and Orthopaedic Surgery, University College Hospital, Division of Surgery and Interventional Science, University College London, London, United Kingdom

JEREMY L. GILBERT, PhD
Department of Bioengineering, Clemson University, Clemson, South Carolina, USA; The Clemson University Medical University of South Carolina Bioengineering Program, Charleston, South Carolina, USA

MARK E. GITTINS, DO
OrthoNeuro, New Albany, Ohio, USA

FABRICE GLOD, MD
Hôpitaux Robert Schuman, Luxembourg-City, Luxembourg

CHRISTOPHER R. GOOD, MD, FACS
Virginia Spine Institute, Reston, Virginia, USA

JEFFREY L. GUM, MD
Norton Leatherman Spine Center, Louisville, Kentucky, USA

FARES S. HADDAD, BSc MD(Res) MCh(Orth), FRCS (Tr&Orth), FFSEM
Department of Trauma and Orthopaedic Surgery, University College Hospital, Division of Surgery and Interventional Science, University College London, London, United Kingdom

EHSAN JAZINI, MD
Virginia Spine Institute, Reston, Virginia, USA

BRENTON R. JENNEWINE, MD
Department of Orthopaedic Surgery and Biomedical Engineering, The University of Tennessee Health Science Center–Campbell Clinic, Campbell Clinic Orthopaedics, Memphis, Tennessee, USA

TODD JONES, BA
Research Assistant, Department of Orthopedic Surgery, Brigham and Women's Hospital, Harvard Medical School, Boston, Massachusetts, USA

BERTRAND P. KAPER, MD
Orthopaedic Specialists of Scottsdale, Scottsdale, Arizona, USA

BABAR KAYANI, BSc (Hons), MBBS, FRCS (Tr&Orth), PhD
Department of Trauma and Orthopaedic Surgery, University College Hospital, London, United Kingdom

JOHN G. KENNEDY, MD, MCh, MMSc, FFSEM, FRCS (Orth)
Chief of Foot and Ankle Surgery, Foot and Ankle Division, Department of Orthopaedic Surgery, NYU Langone Health, New York, New York, USA

MICHAEL A. KURTZ, BS
Department of Bioengineering, Clemson University, Clemson, South Carolina, USA; The Clemson University Medical University of South Carolina Bioengineering Program, Charleston, South Carolina, USA

JEFFREY K. LANGE, MD
Orthopedic Surgeon, Department of Orthopedic Surgery, Brigham and Women's Hospital, Harvard Medical School, Boston, Massachusetts, USA

THOMAS W. McALLISTER, MBBS
Medical Student, Foot and Ankle Division, Department of Orthopaedic Surgery, NYU Langone Health, New York, New York, USA; University of Cambridge School of Clinical Medicine, Cambridge, United Kingdom

GERGO BELA MERKELY, MD
Orthopedic Resident, Department of Orthopedic Surgery, Brigham and Women's Hospital, Harvard Medical School, Boston, Massachusetts, USA

ALEXANDRE BARBIERI MESTRINER, MD
Orthopedic Surgeon, Department of
Orthopedics and Traumatology, Federal
University of Sao Paulo - Paulista, School of
Medicine, Sao Paulo, Brazil

WILLIAM MIHALKO, MD
Department of Orthopaedic Surgery and
Biomedical Engineering, The University of
Tennessee Health Science Center–Campbell
Clinic, Memphis, Tennessee, USA

WILLIAM NELSON, MS
Department of Bioengineering, Clemson
University, Clemson, South Carolina, USA; The
Clemson University Medical University of
South Carolina Bioengineering Program,
Charleston, South Carolina, USA

LINDSAY D. OROSZ, MS, PA-C
National Spine Health Foundation, Reston,
Virginia, USA

RICCI PLASTOW, MBChB, FRCS (Tr&Orth)
Department of Trauma and Orthopaedic
Surgery, University College Hospital, London,
United Kingdom

PIERRE PUTZEYS, MD
Hôpitaux Robert Schuman, Luxembourg-City,
Luxembourg

RAHUL RAI, PhD
Department of Automotive Engineering,
Clemson University, Greenville, South
Carolina, USA

VINAYA RAJAHRAMAN, BS
Department of Orthopedic Surgery, NYU
Langone Health, New York, New York, USA

PIERRE-EMMANUEL SCHWAB, MD
Medical Doctor, Tufts Medical Center, Boston,
Massachusetts, USA

RAN SCHWARZKOPF, MD, MSc
Department of Orthopedic Surgery, NYU
Langone Health, New York, New York, USA

GILES R. SCUDERI, MD
Professor, Department of Orthopedic
Surgery, Northwell Health Orthopedic
Institute, Garden City, New York, USA

BENJAMIN J. SHEFFER, MD
Department of Orthopedic Surgery,
LeBonheur Children's Hospital, Department of
Orthopedic Surgery, The University of
Tennessee Health Science Center–Campbell
Clinic, Memphis, Tennessee, USA; Campbell
Clinic Orthopedics, Germantown, Tennessee,
USA

ITTAI SHICHMAN, MD
Department of Orthopedic Surgery, NYU
Langone Health, New York, New York, USA

PATRICK C. TOY, MD
Department of Orthopaedic Surgery and
Biomedical Engineering, The University of
Tennessee Health Science Center–Campbell
Clinic, Memphis, Tennessee, USA

RAYMOND C. WALLS
Student Researcher, Foot and Ankle Division,
Department of Orthopaedic Surgery, NYU
Langone Health, New York, New York, USA

MAXWELL WEINBERG, MD
Attending Orthopedic Surgeon, Department
of Orthopedic Surgery, Northwell Health
Orthopedic Institute, Garden City, New York,
USA

AUDREY C. WESSINGER
Department of Bioengineering, Clemson
University, Clemson, South Carolina, USA; The
Clemson University Medical University of
South Carolina Bioengineering Program,
Charleston, USA

TAREK YAMOUT, MD
Virginia Spine Institute, Reston, Virginia, USA

RUOYU YANG, PhD
Department of Automotive Engineering,
Clemson University, Greenville, South
Carolina, USA

CONTENTS

Knee and Hip Reconstruction

 Video content accompanies this article at http://www.orthopedic.theclinics.com.

Hip, spine, and pelvis function as a unified kinetic chain. Any spinal pathology,
results in compensatory changes in the other components to accommodate for
the reduced spinopelvic motion. The complex relationship between spinopelvic mobility and component positioning in total hip arthroplasty presents a
challenge in achieving functional implant positioning. Patients with spinal pathology, especially those with stiff spines and little change in sacral slope,
are at high instability risk. In this challenging subgroup, robotic-arm assistance
enables the execution of a patient specific plan, avoiding impingement and
maximizing range of motion; especially utilizing virtual range of motion to
dynamically assess impingement.

One of the primary aims of total knee arthroplasty (TKA) is restoration of the
mechanical axis of the lower limb. Maintenance of the mechanical axis within
3° of neutral has been shown to result in improved clinical results and implant
longevity. Handheld image-free robotic-assisted total knee arthroplasty (HI-
TKA) is a novel way of performing TKA in the era of modern robotic-assisted
TKA. The aim of this study is to assess the accuracy of achieving targeted alignment, component placement, clinical outcomes, as well as patient satisfaction
after HI-TKA.

Background: Robotic-assisted total knee arthroplasty (RA-TKA) has become more popular in the United States. With the significant trend towards performing TKA in outpatient and ambulatory surgery center (ASC) settings, this study was implemented to determine the safety and efficacy of RA-TKA in an ASC. Method: A retrospective review identified 172 outpatient TKAs (86 RA-TKAs and 86 TKAs) performed between January 2020 and January 2021. All surgeries were performed by the same surgeon at the same free-standing ASC. Patients were followed for at least 90 days after surgery; complications, reoperations, readmissions, operative time, and patient-reported outcomes were recorded. Results: In both groups, all patients were successfully discharged home from the ASC on the day of surgery. No differences were noted in overall complications, reoperations, hospital admissions, or delays in discharge. RA-TKA had slightly longer operative times (79 vs 75 min [p = 0.017]) and total length of stay at the ASC (468 vs 412 min [p < 0.0001]) than conventional TKA. No significant differences were noted in outcome scores at 2-, 6-, or 12-week follow-ups. Conclusions: Our results showed that RA-TKA can be successfully implemented in an ASC, with similar outcomes compared with TKA using conventional instrumentation. Initial surgical times were increased secondary to the learning curve of implementing RA-TKA. Long-term follow-up is necessary to determine implant longevity and long-term outcomes.

This review article presents the current state of remote patient monitoring (RPM) in total joint arthroplasty. RPM refers to the use of telecommunication with wearable and implantable technology to assess and treat patients. Several forms of RPM are discussed including telemedicine, patient engagement platforms, wearable devices, and implantable devices. The benefits to patients and physicians are discussed in the context of postoperative monitoring. Insurance coverage and reimbursement of these technologies are reviewed.

Artificial intelligence (AI) is used in the clinic to improve patient care. While the successes illustrate AI's impact, few studies have led to improved clinical outcomes. In this review, we focus on how AI models implemented in nonorthopedic fields of corrosion science may apply to the study of orthopedic alloys. We first define and introduce fundamental AI concepts and models, as well as physiologically relevant corrosion damage modes. We then systematically review the corrosion/AI literature. Finally, we identify several AI models that may be implemented to study fretting, crevice, and pitting corrosion of titanium and cobalt chrome alloys.

The purpose of this study was to determine early survivorship and complication rates associated with the implantation of a new patient-specific unicompartmental knee implant cast from a three-dimensional (3D) printed mold, introduced in 2012. We retrospectively reviewed 92 consecutive patients who underwent unicompartmental knee arthroplasty (UKA) with a patient-specific implant cast from a 3D printed mold between September 2012 and October 2015. The early results of a patient-specific UKA implant were favorable in our cohort, with survivorship free from reoperation of 97% at an average 4.5 years follow-up. Future studies are necessary to investigate the long-term performance of this implant. Survivorship of a patient-specific unicompartmental knee arthroplasty implant cast from a 3D printed mold.

Pediatrics

Current technologies for image guidance navigation and robotic assistance with spinal surgery are improving rapidly with several systems commercially available. Newer machine vision technology has several potential advantages. Limited studies have shown similar outcomes to traditional navigation platforms with decreased intraoperative radiation and time required for registration. However, there are no active robotic arms that can be coupled with machine vision navigation. Further research is necessary to justify the cost, potential increased operative time, and workflow issues but the use of navigation and robotics will only continue to expand given the growing body of evidence supporting their use.

Shoulder and Elbow

Shoulder arthroplasty is a rapidly improving and utilized management for end-stage arthritis that is associated with improved functional outcomes, pain relief, and long-term implant survival. Accurate placement of the glenoid and humeral components is critical for improved outcomes. Traditionally, preoperative planning was limited to radiographs and 2-dimensional computed tomography (CT); however, 3-dimensional CT is becoming more commonly utilized and necessary to understand complex glenoid and humeral deformities. To further increase accurate component placement, intraoperative assistive devices–patient-specific instrumentation, navigation, and mixed reality–minimize malpositioning, increase surgeon accuracy, and maximize fixation. These intraoperative technologies likely represent the future of shoulder arthroplasty.

Foot and Ankle

Video content accompanies this article at http://www.orthopedic.theclinics.com.

Osteochondral lesions of the ankle joint are typically associated with a traumatic etiology and present with ankle pain and swelling. Conservative management yields unsatisfactory results because of the poor healing capacity of the articular cartilage. Smaller lesions (<100 mm^2 or <10 mm) can be treated with less invasive procedures such as arthroscopic debridement, anterograde drilling, scaffold-based therapies, and augmentation with biological adjuvants. For patients with large lesions (>100 mm^2 or >10 mm), cystic lesions, uncontained lesions, or patients who have failed prior bone marrow stimulation, management with autologous osteochondral transplantation is indicated.

Spine

Accurate screw placement is critical to avoid vascular or neurologic complications during spine surgery and to maximize fixation for fusion and deformity correction. Computer-assisted navigation, robotic-guided spine surgery, and augmented reality surgical navigation are currently available technologies that have been developed to improve screw placement accuracy. The advent of multiple generations of new technologies within the past 3 decades has presented surgeons with a diverse array of choices when it comes to pedicle screw placement. Considerations for patient safety and optimal outcomes must be paramount when selecting a technology.

TECHNOLOGICAL ADVANCES

SERIES OF RELATED INTEREST

Foot and Ankle Clinics
https://www.foot.theclinics.com/
Clinics in Sports Medicine
https://www.sportsmed.theclinics.com/
Hand Clinics
https://www.hand.theclinics.com/
Physical Medicine and Rehabilitation Clinics
https://www.pmr.theclinics.com/

PREFACE

Since orthopedic surgery was first performed, innovation has driven technological advancements in the diagnosis and treatment of patients with musculoskeletal injuries. The evolution of computers with Internet and cloud technology, improvements in imaging, and the development of artificial intelligence (AI) and additive manufacturing have created a "paradigm shift" in orthopedic surgery and overall health care. Diagnostic challenges are being met by high-tech improvements in imaging, such as three-dimensional (3D) computerized tomography and four-dimensional MRI. Computer navigation and simulation programs are now assisting with preoperative planning. Robot-assisted surgery has become common in many facilities, playing a crucial role in total joint arthroplasty, spine surgery, and tumor reconstruction. These robotic systems offer better precision and accurate implant placement, resulting in reproducible patient outcomes. Sensor-based technology now allows monitoring of postoperative recovery and rehabilitation after joint replacement, and AI is finding its way from basic science to clinical applications in areas of preoperative risk assessment and image recognition that will aid surgeons in making clinical decisions. Current technology will continue to expand and be incorporated into orthopedic practices, and it is imperative that these new developments be implemented only after a careful study of risks versus benefits as well as costs.

This issue is devoted to these rapidly evolving technologies. It includes articles on robot-assisted total joint replacement of the hip, knee, and shoulder, with findings that suggest improved functional positioning of implants leads to better patient outcomes. These robotic and navigational systems likely represent the future of total joint arthroplasty, and reports indicate they can be done safely and efficiently in ambulatory-surgery settings in select patients. Also gaining traction are telemedicine and remote patient monitoring via wearable or implantable sensors, which are showing promising results especially in total joint rehabilitation.

The integrity and longevity of implants have long been concerns in arthroplasty. Corrosion occurs with metal alloys and can occasionally impair function or adversely affect patients. This is one area where AI can assist by determining the likelihood of that occurring. With translational studies on AI lacking, this issue includes a systematic review of the literature on AI and its use in predicting implant corrosion. Also included is a survivorship study of 3D-printed unicompartmental knee arthroplasties in 92 patients that notes favorable early outcomes with an 8.6% overall complication rate.

The use of robotics has gained a foothold in total joint reconstruction, but the most frequent application is in spine surgery. Two studies published in this issue, one in adult and one in pediatric spine surgery, note that computer navigation increases accuracy of pedicle screw placement and can achieve maximum deformity correction while avoiding vascular or neurologic complications. Decreased radiation exposure to surgeons and minimally invasive surgery application are additional benefits.

Technological advancements have occurred in the field of cartilage repair as well. This issue discusses the treatment of osteochondral lesions of the ankle, including augmentation with biologic adjuvants for small lesions and the use of osteochondral transplantation for large lesions that can be enhanced by using biologic adjuvants.

As always, I thank the authors for their outstanding contributions and hope that readers find these articles useful as they contemplate incorporating newer technologies into their practices.

Frederick M. Azar, MD
Campbell Clinic
Department of Orthopaedic Surgery and
Biomedical Engineering
The University of Tennessee Health Science Center
Memphis, TN, USA

E-mail address:
fazar@campbellclinic.com

Knee and Hip Reconstruction

Functional Component Positioning in Total Hip Arthroplasty and the Role of Robotic-Arm Assistance in Addressing Spinopelvic Pathology

Andreas Fontalis, MD, MSc (Res), MRCS (Eng)[a,b,*],
Pierre Putzeys, MD[c],
Ricci Plastow, MBChB, FRCS (Tr&Orth)[a],
Dia Eldean Giebaly, MBChB, MSc, FRCS (Tr&Orth), eMBA[a,b],
Babar Kayani, MBBS, FRCS (Tr&Orth), PhD[a],
Fabrice Glod, MD[c],
Fares S. Haddad, BSc, MD(Res), MCh(Orth), FRCS (Tr&Orth), FFSEM[a,b]

KEYWORDS

- Robotic-arm assistance • Total hip arthroplasty • Spinal pathology • Spinopelvic stiffness
- Functional component positioning • Functional anteversion • Virtual range of motion
- Impingement

KEY POINTS

- Spinal pathology results in compensatory changes in the other components of the hip–spine–pelvis kinetic chain to accommodate for reduced spinopelvic motion.
- Robotic-arm assistance, especially the latest software incorporating virtual range of motion, enables the execution of individualized component positioning in total hip arthroplasty addressing spinopelvic imbalance.
- "Stuck standing" patients are at risk of posterior dislocation, and options to eliminate this include offset increase and/or increase of inclination and anteversion.
- "Stuck sitting" patients are at risk of anterior dislocation, and options to eliminate this include removal of posterior osteophytes, decreased cup anteversion, increased femoral offset or decreased femoral anteversion.

 Video content accompanies this article at http://www.orthopedic.theclinics.com.

INTRODUCTION

Instability and dislocation constitute one of the most common complications following primary total hip arthroplasty (THA) and the commonest indication for early revision.[1]

Its incidence in the literature ranges between 0% and 5%[2] and a recent, retrospective cohort study reporting the results of 16,186 THAs, revealed an adjusted risk of instability between 0.17% and 1.74%.[3] Multiple factors including

[a] Department of Trauma and Orthopaedic Surgery, University College Hospital, 235 Euston Road, London NW1 2BU, UK; [b] Division of Surgery and Interventional Science, University College London, Gower Street, London WC1E 6BT, UK; [c] Hôpitaux Robert Schuman, 9 Rue Edward Steichen, Luxembourg-City 2540, Luxembourg
* Corresponding author.
E-mail address: andreasfontalis@doctors.org.uk

Orthop Clin N Am 54 (2023) 121–140
https://doi.org/10.1016/j.ocl.2022.11.003
0030-5898/23/© 2022 Elsevier Inc. All rights reserved.

restoration of joint biomechanics, optimization of the soft tissue envelope and preservation of tension are known to play a role in achieving stability in THA. However, the single most important objective is accurate implant positioning, tailored to the phenotype and unique biomechanics of each patient. Suboptimal implant positioning has been associated with polyethylene liner fracture, accelerated wear of the prosthetic components, instability and impingement.[1,4]

HISTORY

Historically, arthroplasty surgeons have used predefined "safe" zones of acetabular version and inclination. In his seminal work, Lewinnek and colleagues[5] described in 1978, one of the most commonly accepted zones of acetabular positioning (5° to 25° of anteversion and 30° to 50° of inclination) based on the analysis of a series of 300 total hip replacements. Authors noted that cups positioned outside this "safe" zone had a fourfold dislocation rate.

Nevertheless, there has been an evolution of ideas beyond this initial description.

Callanan and colleagues[6] designated a modified safe zone with reduced inclination (anteversion 5° to 25° and inclination from 30° to 45°) to accommodate for the steeper cups. He also noted that when manual, free-hand techniques or external alignment guides were used, there was a failure rate of 30% to 75% to achieve the desired cup positioning.[6]

With the advent of new technologies and the evolution of navigation, one of the first attempts to define the functional cup positioning and incorporate spinopelvic parameters was seen by DiGioa and colleagues,[7] who expanded upon the work of Murray and colleagues.[8] As opposed to statically describing the cup inclination and anteversion, DiGioa used lateral spinal radiographs in addition to pelvic and hip radiographs; to correlate these angles to the axis of the body and was the first to take into consideration the hip–spine–pelvis relationship.[9]

This article focuses on providing a comprehensive understanding of spinopelvic parameters and the functional spine–pelvis–hip motion surrounding THA. Furthermore, it aims to delineate the role of robotic-arm assistance in achieving patient-tailored, personalized component positioning in THA. To this end, the paper also incorporates surgical cases and techniques, outlining the challenges posed by abnormal spine–hip–pelvis motion and presents a reproducible workflow to overcome them.

ANATOMY
Normal Spine–Pelvis–Hip Motion

Acquiring an in-depth understanding of the functional relationship between the normal spine–pelvis–hip movement is critical for the arthroplasty surgeon. The pelvis–hip–spine unit constitutes an interchangeable geometric construct that adapts to the body's postural kinetic changes.[10]

When transitioning to a sitting position, the lumbar spine and pelvis have to accommodate the required hip flexion and internal rotation of the femur.[9] This is practically achieved by a posterior tilt of the pelvis and loss of the normal lordotic curvature of the spine, which results in a biological opening of the acetabular cup by increasing functional anteversion and inclination.[9,10] Previous research has shown that for each degree of pelvic tilt, an increase in functional acetabular anteversion of 0.8° should be anticipated.[11] The reported normal value of spinopelvic motion with postural changes is 20° and the respective hip motion is flexion between 55° and 70°.[9,12,13]

Considering the spine–pelvis–hip construct functions as a single unit, one can deduce that the magnitude of spinopelvic mobility is directly related to the necessary hip flexion. For example, in patients with a stiff spinopelvic construct, as there is no posterior rollback; additional hip flexion is needed when sitting and more extension when standing,[14] which in turn increases the impingement risk.[9,15]

In relation to changes occurring in the sagittal plane; in standing position an anterior tilt of the pelvis is observed, whereas the lumbar spine takes its normal lordotic curvature. This change facilitates positioning of the acetabulum over the femoral head and the extension of the hip enables load distribution of the trunk over the pelvis.[9]

SPINOPELVIC PARAMETERS AND DEFINITIONS

The anterior pelvic plane (Fig. 1) is demarcated by the two anterior superior iliac spines (ASIS) and the pubic symphysis, whereas the quantitative assessment of the pelvic tilt is provided by the anterior pelvic plane tilt (APPt). The APPt is the angle created between the two ASIS, the pubic symphysis and a vertical reference line.

Pelvic incidence (PI) was first described by Legaye[16] in 1998 and represents a static measurement of the anterior-to-posterior pelvic dimension that quantitatively defines the

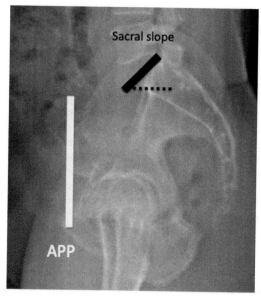

Fig. 1. Lateral radiograph of the lumbar spine showing the anterior pelvic plane and sacral slope.

amount of the lumbar lordosis and pelvic tilt.[16–18] The measurement of the PI allows the evaluation of the functional relationship of the femoral head relative to the spine.[18,19] PI is defined as the angle subtended by a line tangent to the S1 endplate and a line connecting the femoral head to the center of S1 endplate.[20]

The best tool we possess as clinicians to dynamically assess and quantify the spinopelvic motion with postural changes is sacral slope (SS). Sacral slope can be calculated by measuring the angle subtended by a horizontal reference line and a line tangent to the S1 superior endplate (see **Fig. 1**; **Fig. 2**). Specifically, the difference between sitting and standing (ΔSS) is the most accurate representation of the dynamic changes of the pelvis.

The pelvic femoral angle (PFA) is a measure of the femur position relative to the pelvis (180°) and is defined by the angle subtended by a line parallel to the diaphysis of the femur and a second one connecting the center of the femoral head with the center of the S1 endplate.[21]

The acetabular ante-inclination (35°) alludes to the acetabular position in the sagittal plane. Ante-inclination changes with postural changes and pelvic motion and is correlated with the anteversion and inclination of the acetabular cup.

The pelvic tilt can be calculated by the equation: pelvic tilt = pelvic incidence–sacral slope.

The combined anteversion of the femoral stem and acetabular cup in the coronal plane has traditionally been used to provide guidance against impingement. However, the combined sagittal index (CSI), a more sophisticated measure to measure sagittal hip motion and predict stability, has recently been introduced. The CSI is the sum of the ante-inclination and PFA and has been proposed to represent a reliable tool for the functional safe zone to achieve stability in THA.[22–24] A recently published matched cohort study reported that the integration of the CSI led to a reduction in the dislocation risk following THA. Authors also reported that CSI value of <216° (posterior instability and CSI of >244° (anterior instability) in standing position, was one of the strongest predictors of instability.[22]

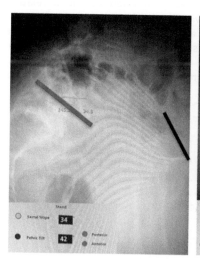
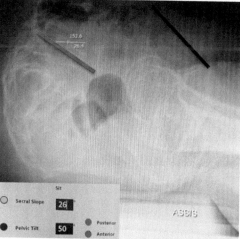

Fig. 2. Figure showing the measurements in standing (*left hand picture*) and sitting (*right hand picture*) of the sacral slope and pelvic tilt.

METHODS TO CLASSIFY SPINOPELVIC MOTION

The most reproducible way to accurately measure the dynamic changes and dynamic motion of the pelvis is the change in sacral slope (ΔSS). Following the influential work of Stefl and colleagues in 2017, it has been established that the normal range of ΔSS from sitting to standing is 11°–29°.[15] A ΔSS < 10 indicates spinopelvic stiffness and in extreme cases where the ΔSS is < 5°; the spinopelvic junction is practically fused, either secondary to surgical intervention or owing to degenerative changes (Fig. 3). Owing to the immobile pelvis there is extreme motion at the hip junction, predisposing individuals to impingement and instability.[25]

On the other end of the spectrum, a ΔSS > 30° signifies a hypermobile spinopelvic construct and is most commonly seen in females and younger patients.[21] Hypermobility at the spinopelvic junction can have a protective role as less hip motion is necessary with postural changes.[26] Conceivably, it has been linked to a low risk of instability.

However, hypermobility can be unbalanced when the spinopelvic construct assumes a kyphotic position when sitting. This involves a sitting sacral slope of <10° and is predominantly encountered in the following conditions. Stiffness of the hips especially ≤50°, which requires an excessive posterior pelvic tilt to offset the loss of hip flexion; patients with neuromuscular disorders and obese patients with a body mass index (BMI) of >40 kg/m² because the mass of the trunk forces the pelvis in increased posterior tilt to achieve balance.[27,28]

As described above, stiffness of the spinopelvic construct can be identified when ΔSS < 10°. Notwithstanding this, delving into the specific patterns of spinal imbalance described by Stefl and colleagues[15] is key to understanding the functional adjustments that need to be made when implanting the components in THA. Stefl and colleagues described three patterns of stiffness contingent on the position in which the spine–pelvis unit is fixed. In patients with ΔSS < 10° and a posterior tilt of the pelvis of > 30°, the spinopelvic construct is considered stiff but not fixed posteriorly or anteriorly.

The second pattern is characterized by a loss of the posterior tilt < 30° when sitting. This pattern is termed "stuck standing" as the pelvis is rigid and fixed in anterior tilt. The functional implication is that there is less biologic opening of the acetabulum when sitting, forcing the hip in more flexion to accommodate the sitting position.

The third pattern is called "stuck sitting" and represents the subset of patients exhibiting no anterior tilt of the pelvis when standing, which is fixed posteriorly (standing sacral tilt <30°).

The functional implication in this situation is the hyperextension of the femur with postural changes to accommodate the standing position. This is represented by an increase of the PFA and puts the patient at risk of posterior impingement (greater trochanter on pelvis and lesser trochanter on ischium)[9] and increased risk of anterior instability.

More recently Vigdorchik and Jerabek proposed the international Hip-Spine classification in THA.[29] This is a simplified classification that encompasses spinal deformity and spinal stiffness.

Spinal deformity is measured by the pelvic incidence minus the lumbar lordotic angle (PI-LL). PI, as described above, is a static morphologic parameter of the anterior-to-posterior pelvic dimension that unveils the functional relationship of the femoral head relative to the pelvis. The lumbar lordotic angle is defined as the angle subtended by two lines at the L1 and S1 superior endplates. The above parameters are key to evaluating spinal balance. With postural changes, any change in the pelvic tilt

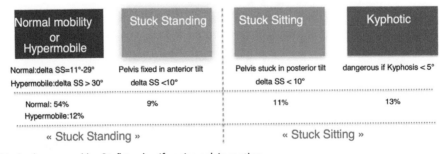

Fig. 3. Method proposed by Stefl to classify spinopelvic motion.

should be inversely related with changes in SS and LL to maintain an upright posture. For an individual to be balanced in the sagittal plane the LL should not be significantly discordant to PI. The concept of PI-LL mismatch as a surrogate for spinal balance in the sagittal plane had previously been introduced by Phan and colleagues.[25] When PI-LL $> 10°$, Vigdorchik[29] described this as a flatback spinal deformity. Subsequently, he categorized patients into those with normal spinal alignment if PI-LL $\pm10°$ (group 1) or a flatback deformity if PI-LL $>10°$ (group 2).

Finally, by coupling spinal deformity (yes or no) and spinal stiffness measured by ΔSS (group A if yes and group B if no), Vigdorchik proposed the following four categories:

1A—normal spinal alignment and normal mobility, 1B—normal spinal alignment and stiffness of the spinopelvic construct, 2A—flatback deformity and normal mobility, and 2B—flatback deformity and stiffness of the spinopelvic construct[29] (**Fig. 4**).

Lastly, another noteworthy classification system is the Bordeaux Classification of Spine–Hip Relations, based on lateral sitting and standing spine radiographs, that entails the measurement of PI, PT, SS and LL.[30]

NATURE OF THE PROBLEM

The relationship between spinal pathology and osteoarthritis of the hip is well-documented in the literature.[31] It has been reported that the prevalence of low back pain is up to 50% in patients undergoing THA.[32]

The ramifications of prior spinal surgery on THA outcomes have been shown in several registry studies from Singapore[33] and the United States[34,35] with patients with prior spinal fusion of 1 to 2 levels exhibiting a dislocation rate of 2.96% and those with 3 to 7 levels a dislocation rate of 4.12%.[33] A more recent systematic review and meta-analysis, encompassing 6 primary studies and a total of 1,456,898 patients showed that

patients with a history of instrumented lumbar fusion had higher dislocation and revision rates.[36]

However, it should not be forgotten that patients can have a stiff spine and abnormal motion in the lower kinetic chain without necessarily having undergone an instrumented fusion.[37,38] This is eloquently shown by Vigdorchik and colleagues[38] who found that out of the 6340 patients included in the study, 6% had a decreased lumbar flexion (defined as $\leq 20°$); out of which only 19% had an instrumented fusion. At a different angle, only 32% of the patients with an instrumented fusion had a lumbar flexion $\leq 20°$.[38]

Restoring the hip offset has well recognized biomechanical advantages including an increase in the abductor moment arm and decreased joint reaction forces. However, a strong relationship between offset and instability has yet to be established.

Theoretically, increasing the offset could confer advantageous results in patients with a stiff spine as the trochanter is positioned further away from the pelvis, hence reducing the risk of impingement. In a large retrospective study of 12,365 patients, Vigdorchik and colleagues[39] reported that within the subset of patients sustaining a dislocation ($N = 51$), 96% had a standard-offset stem implanted. Furthermore, authors utilized an impingement model and found there was a 5° added range of motion (ROM) until impingement was observed for every 1 mm offset increase.[39] In addition, Heckman and colleagues[40] showed that under-restoration of the hip offset was more prevalent among patients with instability, whereas large diameter heads were more common among stable hips.

Lastly, there is mounting evidence debunking the safety of the traditional Lewinnek zone. Abdel and colleagues[2] conducted a retrospective review of 206 patients that sustained a dislocation over a 10 year period and discovered that the inclination and anteversion of the acetabular component was within the "safe zone" in 84% and 69% of the hips respectively.

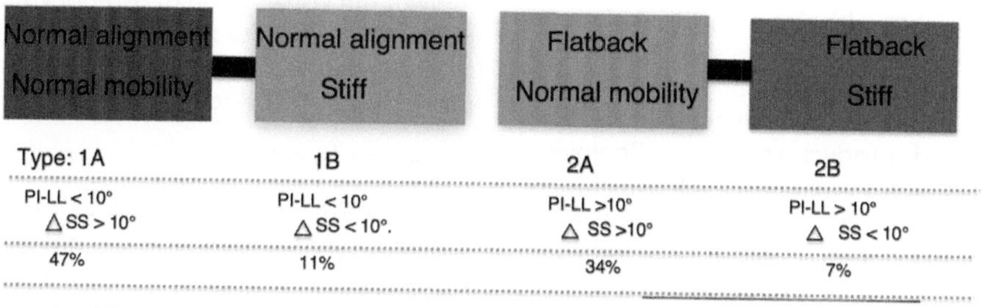

Normal alignment Normal mobility	Normal alignment Stiff	Flatback Normal mobility	Flatback Stiff
Type: 1A	1B	2A	2B
PI-LL < 10° $\triangle$ SS > 10°	PI-LL < 10° $\triangle$ SS < 10°.	PI-LL >10° $\triangle$ SS >10°	PI-LL > 10° $\triangle$ SS < 10°
47%	11%	34%	7%

Fig. 4. International hip–spine classification proposed by Vigdorchik and colleagues.

THE ROLE OF ROBOTIC-ARM ASSISTANCE

The advent of advanced surgical technologies such as computer navigation and robotic arm-assistance has enabled the accurate reproducibility of the preoperative plan and has brought to the fore the concept of personalized, functional component positioning in THA.

The most commonly used robotic system at present is the MAKO system,[41] an active constrained system.[42] The workflow commences with the segmentation of the CT and the creation of a three-dimensional plan delivered to the surgeon to optimize precision and component implantation, incorporating spinopelvic parameters. The latest version of the software (MAKO 4.0) includes a virtual range of motion (vROM) tool that enables real time, intraoperative feedback and visualization of impingement, as well as the impact of changes in component orientation. There is good quality data suggesting that robotic arm-assisted THA is associated with better reproducibility in relation to cup positioning and leads to more accurate restoration of the native center of rotation, offset and leg-length.[43–46]

In this article we aim to present a reproducible workflow, utilizing robotic-arm assistance to achieve personalized component positioning, deliver individualized THA and tackle the challenges emerging from spinopelvic pathology.

Preoperative planning

"If you fail to prepare, then prepare to fail" is an adage worth remembering within orthopedic surgery. Preoperative planning in THA is the cornerstone of good surgical practice, which affords the benefit of delineating the anatomy and respecting the individual phenotype of the patient.

The key benefit of utilizing the robotic software is the detailed preoperative planning of implant positioning in relation to the 3-dimensional anatomy of the hip joint, that has not been possible with 2-dimensional radiographic imaging in the past. Significant dysplasia can be scrutinized and co-morbidities such as spinal pathology and previous trauma can be taken into account when planning the acetabular cup position and stem version. The starting position for the acetabular cup is 40° inclination and 20° anteversion. At this stage it is essential to involve the designated product specialist. Conjointly with the operating surgeon they will dynamically evaluate the presence of impingement and ROM and modify the angles in accordance with the native anatomy and surgeon preference.

Preoperative workflow

Preoperative sitting and standing lateral lumbar spine radiographs[37] allow assessment of the spinal mobility (Fig. 5).

Subsequently, rotating the 3D pelvis image with the cup superimposed enables the assessment of several positional parameters. It is key for the arthroplasty surgeon to consider all the points below:

- *Cup center of rotation*

The cup position with the center of rotation highlighted as a green dot can be compared with the native femoral head center of rotation. The transverse view should be utilized to inspect the medio-lateral position of the cup and whether the chosen size achieves satisfactory bony coverage. Each surgeon will have a different philosophy on whether to keep the center of rotation lateral for bone preservation and restore native offset or medialize to gain better cup coverage and osteointegration.

- *Cup version*

It is essential to visualize there is no anterior cup prominence which may irritate the psoas tendon causing groin pain post-operatively. Furthermore, in dysplastic acetabuli where the posterior wall is deficient, it is possible to appreciate the amount of cup uncovered posteriorly.

- *Stem size*

This can be accurately judged in three planes and pre-plan the neck cut to restore leg length and native offset.

- *Stem version*

The native version is calculated and if found to be excessively anteverted or even retroverted then plans for changing offset can be made preoperatively with canal preparation or alternative cemented or modular stems.

- *Osteophytes*

With the visualization of osteophytes, the surgeon can appreciate the cup position in relation to these and the potential need for excision to prevent implant or bony impingement.

- *Leg length*

This is accurately measured using bony landmarks on the CT scan. The designated product specialist and the surgeon should ensure the

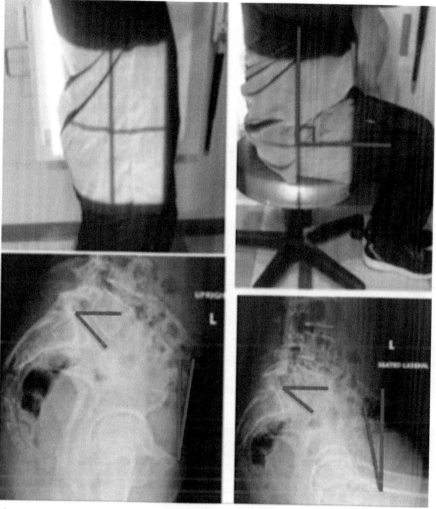

Fig. 5. Lumbar spine lateral standing and sitting radiographs. The anterior superior iliac spine and pubic symphysis need to be included to allow the anterior pelvic tilt angle to be calculated with the MAKO 4.0 software. Alternatively, the sacral slope can be calculated (*red lines*).

bony landmarks used are accurate (examples include the tear drop and lesser trochanter).

In Video 1 and the figures below, we present a stepwise approach in a patient with stiff spinopelvic construct and illustrate the changes that had to be made at the preoperative planning stage to avoid impingement.

- The first step is to import the spinopelvic measurements obtained by the sitting and standing lateral radiographs into the software and appreciate the motion of the spinopelvic construct. The supine pelvic tilt can also be calculated from the CT scan with the help of the software at this stage. The operating surgeon and designated product specialist should ensure all the pelvic landmarks are correctly identified (ASIS, pubic tubercle). We used the sacral slope as a surrogate and the difference with postural changes ΔSS was only 8°; hence, the patient was classified as having a stiff spine (Fig. 6A, B)
- The next step is to correctly identify conjointly with the designated product specialist, the anatomical landmarks to allow leg length measurement (tear drop and lesser trochanter in this case) (Fig. 6C).
- The starting position for the acetabular cup is 40° inclination and 20° anteversion. The position is then assessed in all three planes (transverse, coronal, and sagittal) to ensure restoration of the center of rotation, adequate coverage, avoid prominence and evaluate the posterior wall (Fig. 7A–C).

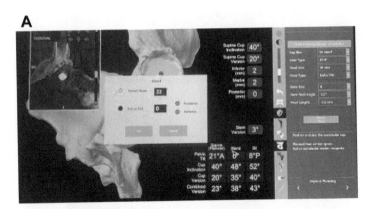

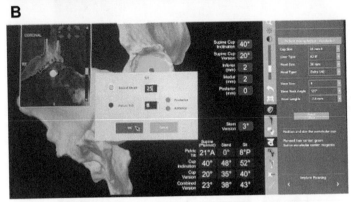

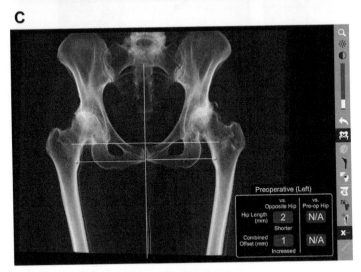

Fig. 6. (A) Importing sacral slope in standing. (B) Importing sacral slope in sitting. The difference ΔSS is only 8°, hence raising awareness for the presence of stiff spinopelvic construct. (C) Preoperative plan with no implant superimposed. The tear drops and lesser trochanters have been used as landmarks to allow leg length measurements.

- Moving on to the stem positioning, the surgeon should look at the 2-dimensional predicted post-operative appearance and focus on the stem size, offset and leg length. Choosing the right stem size without underfilling the canal or compromising the calcar is key. Furthermore, any valgus or varus malalignment can be corrected (Fig. 8A).

In this case we noted that combined offset was decreased and given the case involved a stiff spinopelvic construct it was essential to preserve this. Hence, it was anticipated that we would have to lateralize the cup and/or use a 0 mm head.

- The next step is to evaluate the stem version by looking at the transverse and sagittal views. The transverse view is

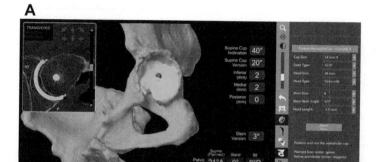

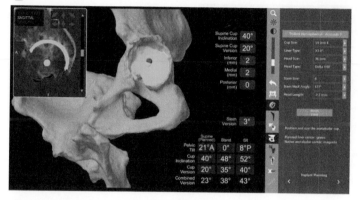

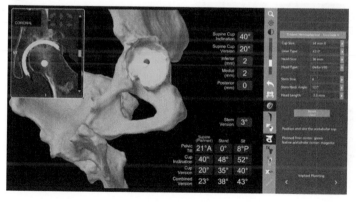

Fig. 7. (A) Assessment of the cup position in the transverse plane. (B) Assessment of the cup position in the sagittal plane. (C) Assessment of the cup position in the coronal plane.

principally helpful to assess the native version and the appropriate amount of anteversion that has to be applied (Fig. 8B, C).

- The evolution of robotic technology and the introduction of the latest software 4.0 has led to a ground-breaking feature, allowing the surgeon to assess the pelvis mechanics and analyze hip-spine movement. Where the real power of the software lies, is the dynamic, real-time assessment of impingement. The hip is tested in 110°

flexion and 40° internal rotation. In this case, we noted that both bone-on-bone and prosthetic impingement were evident (Fig. 9A, B).

- Considering the presence of impingement and the fact combined offset was decreased by 2 mm, we proceeded to lateralizing the cup by 1 mm (Fig. 10A). As seen in Figure this resulted in elimination of the majority of bone-on-bone impingement, however

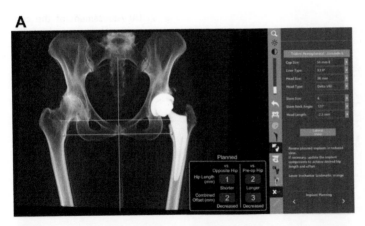

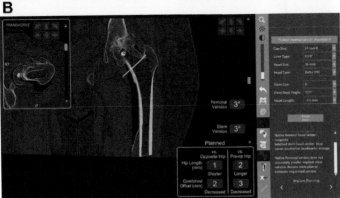

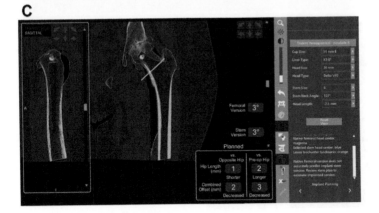

Fig. 8. (A) Predicted postoperative radiographic appearance. (B) Transverse view of the stem, enabling the assessment of native anteversion and the appropriate anteversion of the stem. (C) Sagittal view of the stem during preoperative planning.

the prosthetic impingement persisted as expected (Fig. 10B).

- Despite the changes, intraprosthetic impingement was still evident. To address this, we modified the orientation of the cup by adding 44° inclination and 22° anteversion (Fig. 12A, B). With the above changes, we also avoided decreasing the offset, a very important surgical target particularly in stiff patients.

Procedural Approach

Fig. 13 outlines our intraoperative workflow in robotic-arm assisted THA, also used to address the challenging cases of spinopelvic stiffness. The femoral stem preparation is carried out first to allow as much correction as possible on the stem version. If the preoperative plan highlights excessive anteversion or retroversion of the femoral neck, then this can be addressed. If there is still a problem with impingement, the

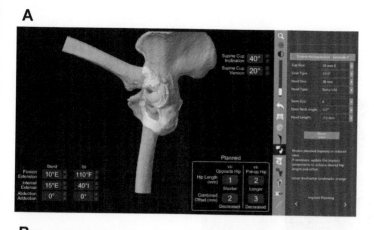

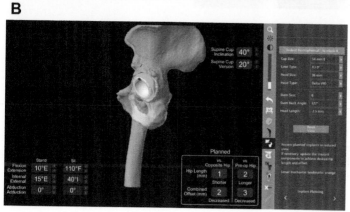

Fig. 9. (A) Virtual ROM tool allowing the identification of impingement and type. (B) Virtual ROM tool after removing the femur for better visualization of the impingement.

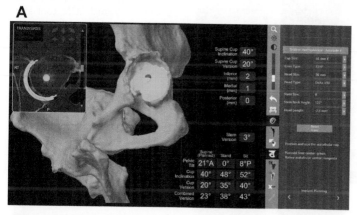

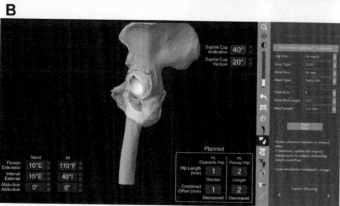

Fig. 10. (A) Lateralization of the cup by 1 mm to increase offset and eliminate bone-on-bone impingement. (B) Testing for impingement after lateralization of the cup. We noted that even after lateralizing the cup there was still a minor degree of bone-on-bone impingement and to eliminate this we opted for a 0 mm head (Fig. 11).

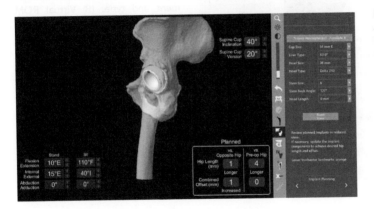

Fig. 11. Virtual ROM after selecting a 0 mm head, where persistent intraprosthetic impingement is evident.

stem can still be changed to a cemented stem or modular stem. If the acetabulum is prepared first, then the shell may have to be removed later in the procedure if more version or inclination is needed.

Femoral registration begins with placing a screw into the greater trochanter for the femoral array and a further checkpoint into the trochanter as seen in Figs. 14 and 15, and Video 2. The surgeon then performs registration of the femur by placing a pointed probe onto several areas of the femur highlighted on the screen. This confirms the CT scan 3D model matches the patient and the infra-red sensors can pick up the position of the femur before any cuts are made.

Combined Anteversion

Once the femur is prepared the combined anteversion is calculated on screen. Fig. 16 shows the screen and highlights the inclination and

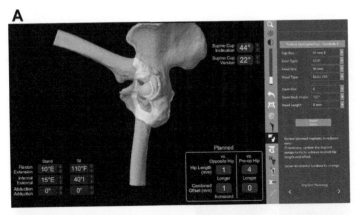

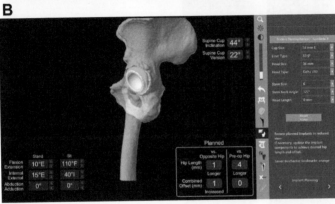

Fig. 12. (A). Virtual ROM tool after increasing the inclination and anteversion. (B) Virtual ROM tool after removing the femur, showing no impingement after increasing the inclination and anteversion.

Workflow

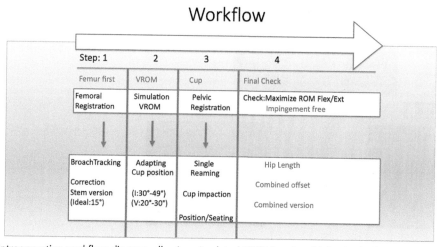

Step: 1	2	3	4
Femur first	VROM	Cup	Final Check
Femoral Registration	Simulation VROM	Pelvic Registration	Check:Maximize ROM Flex/Ext Impingement free
BroachTracking Correction Stem version (Ideal:15°)	Adapting Cup position (I:30°-49°) (V:20°-30°)	Single Reaming Cup impaction Position/Seating	Hip Length Combined offset Combined version

Fig. 13. Intraoperative workflow diagram allowing simulated VROM and multiple checks for impingement.

version angles changing from standing to sitting as described earlier. This is a key feature introduced in the new robotic software allowing to assess pelvic mechanics and dynamically visualize the cup position when seated and standing. This enables the arthroplasty surgeon to identify any case-specific challenges and pre-empt any difficulties.

ADDRESSING THE SPINOPELVIC CHALLENGE WITH ROBOTICS

The following case illustrates how robotic-arm assistance can be utilized in practice to tackle the challenge of spinopelvic stiffness. This case presents a 72-year-old patient with previous spinal fusion surgery and stiff spine classified as stuck sitting or hip spine classification 2B. Figs. 17–20 highlight the workflow to prevent posterior impingement in standing position with external rotation of the hip and potential anterior dislocation. Implant-on-implant impingement was present and decreasing the cup version was necessary in this scenario (see Fig. 19). Bone-on-bone impingement was also present in standing position and dictated the removal of posterior osteophytes as highlighted in (see Fig. 20).

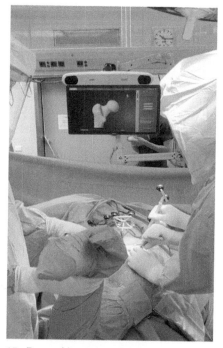

Fig. 14. Position of the femoral and pelvic arrays. The yellow circle highlights the broach within the femoral canal with the probe checking the stem version.

Fig. 15. Femoral bone registration.

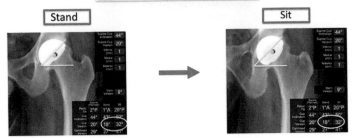

	Supine (Planned)	Stand	Sit
Pelvic Tilt	2°P	1°A	20°P
Cup Inclination	44°	43°	50°
Cup Version	20°	18°	32°
Combined Version	29°	27°	41°

Fig. 16. Showing the significant increase in cup inclination and version when sitting from a standing position.

BAIL OUT OPTIONS

The last resort in cases of stiff spines is dual mobility cups, which is currently the most common options for spinal disease patients. The smaller diameter cup sizes however, with the inner diameter 28 mm head, do not provide a significantly larger range of movement or clearance from bony impingement over the 36 mm head. It is only in the larger acetabular cups where the benefit is seen. As the long-term survivorship of this implant in younger patients with spinal stiffness is not yet established, it should be attempted to use the less constrained cup in these cases if possible.

OUTCOMES

Vigdorchik and colleagues[29] in their influential study introducing and validating the international hip-spine Classification, used personalized, patient-specific inclination and anteversion targets based on risk stratification. Patients considered at high risk for dislocation due to spinal deformity and/or stiffness (classified as 1B, 2A, and 2B), underwent THA using a high-risk protocol. This

72 year old female - Left hip

- Partial fusion L5-S1
- Scoliosis
- Lumbar degenerative disc disease, facet spondylosis
- Large posterior Pelvic Tilt(>13°)and Spinal Stiffness: « Stuck Sitting »
- Hip-Spine Classification:2B—> increasing anterior instability risk

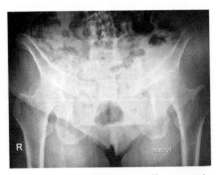
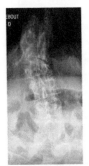
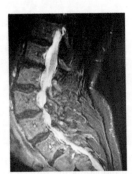

Fig. 17. Case scenario of stuck sitting stiff spine with anterior dislocation risk.

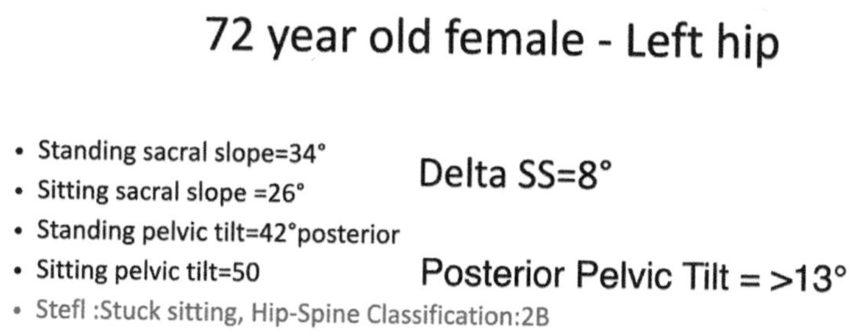

72 year old female - Left hip

- Standing sacral slope=34°
- Sitting sacral slope =26°
- Standing pelvic tilt=42°posterior
- Sitting pelvic tilt=50
- Stefl :Stuck sitting, Hip-Spine Classification:2B

Delta SS=8°

Posterior Pelvic Tilt = >13°

Fig. 18. Showing the pelvis is stuck with a posterior tilt rather than anterior tilt as normal in standing position. The delta slope change is only 8°, representing significant stiffness in the spine.

Standing E10°/ER15°

- **Implant to Implant impingement at the posterior border**
- **Correction of cup anteversion from 24° to 22°**

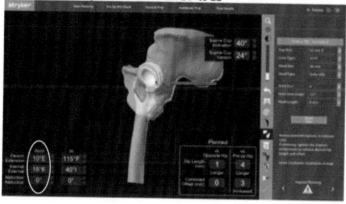

Fig. 19. Illustration of posterior impingement (*red area*) in standing with external rotation at 15°. The cup version was reduced to eliminate this.

Bone on Bone impingement in Standing

- Removal of posterior osteophytes to avoid bone to bone impingement

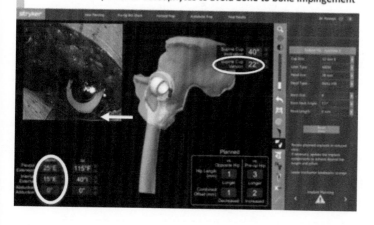

Fig. 20. Highlighting the need for removal of posterior osteophytes to prevent bone-on-bone impingement and potential anterior dislocation.

Table 1
Results and characteristics of large studies reporting outcomes following functional or personalized acetabular cup positioning

Author and Date	Patient Cohort	Study Type	Methodological Features	Interventions	Outcomes	Key Results
Vigdorchik et al,[29] 2021	3,777 patients prospectively undergoing THA by three surgeons	Prospective multicenter study (level III evidence)	Participants categorized according to the international Hip-Spine Classification in THA	Patient-specific inclination and anteversion targets for each group based on spinopelvic measurements	Survivorship free of dislocation	Survivorship free of dislocation at five years was 99.2% with a 0.8% dislocation rate
Esposito et al,[48] 2018	1000 patients who underwent post-operative biplanar spine-to-ankle lateral radiographs in standing and sitting position 1 year following THA	Prospective Cross sectional study (level IV evidence)	Posterior approach Imageless optical navigation used	Standing and sitting radiographs at 1 year Spinopelvic alignment parameters (sacral slope, lumbar lordosis, and proximal femur angle)	Acetabular component position Dislocation Spinopelvic alignment	92% (11 of 12) of the patients sustaining a dislocation had a surgical spine fusion or lumbar multi-level degenerative disc disease
Vigdorchik et al,[47] 2019	111 patients undergoing revision THA for recurrent instability	Retrospective case control study (level III evidence)	Participants categorized according to the Hip-Spine Classification in revision THA Mean follow up was 2.8 years Posterior Approach	Functional position of the spine utilized to inform component positioning in revision THA (protocol) Versus a matched 1:1 group of 111 revisions performed not using the protocol.	Survivorship free of dislocation	Survival free of dislocation at two years was 97% in the protocol group versus 84% in the control group

| Sharma et al,[49] 2021 | 1500 consecutive primary THAs | Retrospective cohort (level IV evidence) | Direct Anterior or posterior approach 2-year follow up 4 sagittal functional x-rays taken (supine, standing, flex-seated, and step-up) Low-dose CT scan to capture the individual's bony hip anatomy and soft tissue landmarks Pelvic tilt, pelvic incidence, and lumbar flexion angles measured | Patient specific femoral and acetabular component templating utilizing the OPS computer bases software program. Laser handle guides component positioning intraoperatively | Implant positioning Dislocations | Only 6/1500 (0.4%) of all implanted cups dislocated postoperatively, all dislocations were in cups within the Lewinnek's zone Only 56% of hips that underwent dynamic preoperative acetabular cup planning were within the Lewinnek's zone |

included preservation of offset using a 36 mm component if possible; and using a dual mobility (DM) component in all group 2B patients. Survivorship free of dislocation at five years was 99.2%, with only 0.8% of patients having sustained a dislocation.[29]

In patients with recurrent instability following THA, Vigdorchik and colleagues[47] also described a similar algorithm, the Hip-Spine Classification in Revision THA, to assess the functional position of the spine. This was subsequently used to inform decision making in revision THA, resulting in a significantly decreased risk of further instability compared with a control group. Authors reported a two-year 97% survival free of dislocation compared with 84% in the control group following treatment.

Esposito and colleagues[48] examined a consecutive series of 1000 patients who underwent post-operative biplanar lateral radiographs in standing and sitting positions 1 year following THAs. Patients experiencing a dislocation had significantly less spine flexion (mean 14° vs 23°, $P < .001$), less change in pelvic tilt (mean change in sacral slope 9° vs 17°, $P = .01$), and more hip flexion (72° vs 65°, $P = .001$) from standing to sitting positions compared with patients with normal spinal mobility.[48]

Sharma and colleagues[49] compared preoperative acetabular cup parameters using a novel dynamic imaging sequence to the safe zone suggested by Lewinnek. They found that only 56% of hips that underwent dynamic preoperative acetabular cup planning were within the Lewinnek's zone. Of the 1500-patient cohort, there were 6 dislocations (0.4%); all occurring in cups positioned within the Lewinnek's zone.[49] The low dislocation rate with dynamic imaging seen in their cohort further supports the claim that the only true "safe zones" are functional zones (Table 1).

SUMMARY

Robotic-arm assisted THA is a valuable tool in the surgical armamentarium, especially in the challenging subset of spinal pathology patients in whom achievement of the desired offset, leg-length and component positioning is key to avoid impingement. The evolution of robotic technology has recently enabled the assessment of virtual ROM; a feature with immense potential in achieving functional component positioning and tackling the challenge of reduced spinopelvic motion.

Acquiring a comprehensive understanding of spinopelvic parameters and delving into the specific patterns of spinal imbalance is of paramount importance for the arthroplasty surgeon.

Furthermore, the thinking in 3D planning involved in robotic THA can help surgeons to better understand future goals and can serve as a valuable training tool.

Finally, there is mounting evidence to suggest that the leap from historical "safe zones" to functional ones, has resulted in reducing the dislocation risk and better radiological outcomes. To this end, robotic technology offers an avenue to segment the procedure, analyze ample data and redefine the accepted zones of component positioning.

CLINICS CARE POINTS

- Acquiring a comprehensive understanding of the functional spine–pelvis–hip relationship is of paramount importance for the arthroplasty surgeon. It constitutes an interchangeable geometric construct that functionally adapts to postural kinetic changes.

- It should not be forgotten that spinal surgery is not a prerequisite for spinal stiffness, and abnormal motion in the lower kinetic chain can be present without prior instrumented fusion.

- There is mounting evidence that a large proportion of dislocations occur within the historically perceived "safe zones".

- Robotic-arm assistance is a valuable tool and a pragmatic solution to address the challenge of functional component positioning in patients with spinal pathology, offering reproducible and accurate results.

- "Stuck standing" patients are at risk of posterior instability, and offset increase and/or adding more inclination and anteversion may be necessary.

- "Stuck sitting" patients are at risk of anterior instability, and options include removing posterior osteophytes, decreasing cup anteversion, or increasing femoral offset.

ACKNOWLEDGMENTS

The authors would like to acknowledge Ms Melanie Maligsay for her support and help with the robotic software and figures. A. Fontalis would like to acknowledge the financial support provided by the Freemasons'

Royal Arch Fellowship with support from the Arthritis Research Trust.

SUPPLEMENTARY DATA

Supplementary data related to this article can be found online at https://doi.org/10.1016/j.ocl.2022.11.003.

REFERENCES

1. Fontalis A, Berry DJ, Shimmin A, et al. Prevention of early complications following total hip replacement. SICOT-J 2021;7:61.

2. Abdel MP, von Roth P, Jennings MT, et al. What Safe Zone? The Vast Majority of Dislocated THAs Are Within the Lewinnek Safe Zone for Acetabular Component Position. Clin Orthop Relat Res 2016;474(2):386–91.

3. Fleischman AN, Tarabichi M, Magner Z, et al. Mechanical Complications Following Total Hip Arthroplasty Based on Surgical Approach: A Large, Single-Institution Cohort Study. J Arthroplasty 2019;34(6):1255–60.

4. Khan M, Della Valle CJ, Jacofsky DJ, et al. Early postoperative complications after total hip arthroplasty: current strategies for prevention and treatment. Instr Course Lect 2015;64:337–46.

5. Lewinnek GE, Lewis JL, Tarr R, et al. Dislocations after total hip-replacement arthroplasties - PubMed. J Bone Jt Surg Am 1978;60(2):217–20.

6. Callanan MC, Jarrett B, Bragdon CR, et al. The John Charnley Award: risk factors for cup malpositioning: quality improvement through a joint registry at a tertiary hospital. Clin Orthop Relat Res 2011;469(2):319–29.

7. DiGioia AM, Jaramaz B, Blackwell M, et al. The Otto Aufranc Award. Image guided navigation system to measure intraoperatively acetabular implant alignment. Clin Orthop Relat Res 1998;355(355):8–22.

8. Murray DW. The definition and measurement of acetabular orientation. J Bone Joint Surg Br 1993;75(2):228–32.

9. Heckmann N, Trasolini NA, Stefl M, et al. The Effect of Spinopelvic Motion on Implant Positioning and Hip Stability Using the Functional Safe Zone of THR. Pers Hip Knee Jt Replace 2020;133–42. https://doi.org/10.1007/978-3-030-24243-5_1.

10. Klemt C, Limmahakhun S, Bounajem G, et al. Effect of postural changes on in vivo pelvic tilt and functional component anteversion in total hip arthroplasty patients with lumbar disc degenerations. Bone Joint J 2020;102 B(11):1505–10.

11. Wan Z, Malik A, Jaramaz B, et al. Imaging and navigation measurement of acetabular component position in THA. Clin Orthop Relat Res 2009;467(1):32–42.

12. Larkin B, van Holsbeeck M, Koueiter D, et al. What is the impingement-free range of motion of the asymptomatic hip in young adult males? Clin Orthop Relat Res 2015;473(4):1284–8.

13. Lazennec JY, Charlot N, Gorin M, et al. Hip-spine relationship: a radio-anatomical study for optimization in acetabular cup positioning. Surg Radiol Anat 2004;26(2):136–44.

14. Bracey DN, Hegde V, Shimmin AJ, et al. Spinopelvic mobility affects accuracy of acetabular anteversion measurements on cross-table lateral radiographs. Bone Joint J 2021;103-B(7):59–65.

15. Stefl M, Lundergan W, Heckmann N, et al. Spinopelvic mobility and acetabular component position for total hip arthroplasty. Bone Joint J 2017;99-B(1 Supple A):37–45.

16. Legaye J, Duval-Beaupère G, Hecquet J, et al. Pelvic incidence: a fundamental pelvic parameter for three-dimensional regulation of spinal sagittal curves. Eur Spine J 1998;7(2):99–103.

17. Kleeman-Forsthuber L, Vigdorchik JM, Pierrepont JW, et al. Pelvic incidence significance relative to spinopelvic risk factors for total hip arthroplasty instability. Bone Joint J 2022;104(3):352–8.

18. Heckmann N, Tezuka T, Bodner RJ, et al. Functional Anatomy of the Hip Joint. J Arthroplasty 2021;36(1):374–8.

19. Iwasa M, Ando W, Uemura K, et al. Pelvic incidence is not associated with the development of hip osteoarthritis. Bone Joint J 2021;103-B(11):1656–61.

20. Czubak-Wrzosek M, Nitek Z, Sztwiertnia P, et al. Pelvic incidence and pelvic tilt can be calculated using either the femoral heads or acetabular domes in patients with hip osteoarthritis. Bone Joint J 2021;103-B(8):1345–50.

21. Ike H, Dorr LD, Trasolini N, et al. Current concepts review spine-pelvis-hip relationship in the functioning of a total hip replacement. J Bone Jt Surg - Am 2018;100(18):1606–15.

22. Grammatopoulos G, Falsetto A, Sanders E, et al. Integrating the Combined Sagittal Index Reduces the Risk of Dislocation Following Total Hip Replacement. J Bone Jt Surg - Am 2022;104(5):397–411.

23. Heckmann N, McKnight B, Stefl M, et al. Late dislocation following total hip arthroplasty: Spinopelvic imbalance as a causative factor. J Bone Jt Surg - Am 2018;100(21):1845–53.

24. Bodner RJ. The Functional Mechanics of the Acetabular Component in Total Hip Arthroplasty. J Arthroplasty 2022. https://doi.org/10.1016/J.ARTH.2022.05.017.

25. Phan D, Bederman SS, Schwarzkopf R. The influence of sagittal spinal deformity on anteversion of the acetabular component in total hip arthroplasty. Bone Joint J 2015;97-B(8):1017–23.

26. Sculco PK, Windsor EN, Jerabek SA, et al. Preoperative spinopelvic hypermobility resolves following total hip arthroplasty. Bone Joint J 2021;103 B(12): 1766–73.

27. Esposito CI, Miller TT, Kim HJ, et al. Does Degenerative Lumbar Spine Disease Influence Femoroacetabular Flexion in Patients Undergoing Total Hip Arthroplasty? Clin Orthop Relat Res 2016; 474(8):1788–97.

28. Ike H, Dorr LD, Trasolini N, et al. Spine-Pelvis-Hip Relationship in the Functioning of a Total Hip Replacement. J Bone Joint Surg Am 2018;100(18): 1606–15.

29. Vigdorchik JM, Sharma AK, Buckland AJ, et al. 2021 Otto Aufranc Award: A simple Hip-Spine Classification for total hip arthroplasty. Bone Joint J 2021; 103-B(7):17–24.

30. Zagra L, Benazzo F, Dallari D, et al. Current concepts in hip–spine relationships: making them practical for total hip arthroplasty. EFORT Open Rev 2022;7(1):59–69.

31. Mononen H, Sund R, Halme J, et al. Following total hip arthroplasty: femoral head component diameter of 32 mm or larger is associated with lower risk of dislocation in patients with a prior lumbar fusion. Bone Joint J 2020;102(8):1003–9.

32. Parvizi J, Pour AE, Hillibrand A, et al. Back pain and total hip arthroplasty: A prospective natural history study. Clin Orthop Relat Res 2010;468(5):1325–30.

33. Buckland AJ, Puvanesarajah V, Vigdorchik J, et al. Dislocation of a primary total hip arthroplasty is more common in patients with a lumbar spinal fusion. Bone Jt J 2017;99B(5):585–91.

34. Loh JLM, Jiang L, Chong HC, et al. Effect of Spinal Fusion Surgery on Total Hip Arthroplasty Outcomes: A Matched Comparison Study. J Arthroplasty 2017;32(8):2457–61.

35. Salib CG, Reina N, Perry KI, et al. Lumbar fusion involving the sacrum increases dislocation risk in primary total hip arthroplasty. Bone Joint J 2019; 101 B(2):198–206.

36. An VVG, Phan K, Sivakumar BS, et al. Prior Lumbar Spinal Fusion is Associated With an Increased Risk of Dislocation and Revision in Total Hip Arthroplasty: A Meta-Analysis. J Arthroplasty 2018;33(1): 297–300.

37. Ransone M, Fehring K, Fehring T. Standardization of lateral pelvic radiograph is necessary to predict spinopelvic mobility accurately. Bone Joint Journa 2020;102(7):41–6.

38. Vigdorchik JM, Sharma AK, Dennis DA, et al. The Majority of Total Hip Arthroplasty Patients With a Stiff Spine Do Not Have an Instrumented Fusion. J Arthroplasty 2020;35(6):S252–4.

39. Vigdorchik JM, Sharma AK, Elbuluk AM, et al. High Offset Stems Are Protective of Dislocation in High-Risk Total Hip Arthroplasty. J Arthroplasty 2021; 36(1):210–6.

40. Heckmann ND, Chung BC, Wier JR, et al. The Effect of Hip Offset and Spinopelvic Abnormalities on the Risk of Dislocation Following Total Hip Arthroplasty. J Arthroplasty 2022;37(7S):S546–51.

41. Zhang J, Ng N, Scott CEH, et al. Robotic arm-assisted versus manual unicompartmental knee arthroplasty : a systematic review and meta-analysis of the MAKO robotic system. Bone Joint J 2022;104-B(5):541–8.

42. Fontalis A, Epinette J-A, Thaler M, et al. Advances and innovations in total hip arthroplasty. SICOT-J 2021;7:26.

43. Emara AK, Zhou G, Klika AK, et al. Is there increased value in robotic arm-assisted total hip arthroplasty? Bone Joint J 2021;103-B(9): 1488–96.

44. Kayani B, Konan S, Thakrar RR, et al. Assuring the long-term total joint arthroplasty: a triad of variables. Bone Joint J 2019;101-B(1_Supple_A):11–8.

45. Kayani B, Konan S, Huq SS, et al. The learning curve of robotic-arm assisted acetabular cup positioning during total hip arthroplasty. Hip Int 2021;31(3): 311–9.

46. Ng N, Gaston P, Simpson PM, et al. Robotic arm-assisted versus manual total hip arthroplasty. Bone Joint J 2021;103-B(6):1009–20.

47. Vigdorchik J, Jerabek SA, Mayman DJ, et al. Evaluation of the spine is critical in the workup of recurrent instability after total hip arthroplasty. Bone Joint J 2019;101-B(7):817–23.

48. Esposito CI, Carroll KM, Sculco PK, et al. Total hip arthroplasty patients with fixed spinopelvic alignment are at higher risk of hip dislocation. J Arthroplasty 2018;33(5):1449–54.

49. Sharma AK, Cizmic Z, Dennis DA, et al. Low dislocation rates with the use of patient specific "Safe zones" in total hip arthroplasty. J Orthop 2021;27: 41–8.

Clinical, Radiographic, and Patient-Reported Outcomes Associated with a Handheld Image-free Robotic-Assisted Surgical System in Total Knee Arthroplasty

Ittai Shichman, MD[a,1], Vinaya Rajahraman, BS[a,1],
James Chow, MD[b], David W. Fabi, MD[c],
Mark E. Gittins, DO[d], Joseph E. Burkhardt, DO[e],
Bertrand P. Kaper, MD[f], Ran Schwarzkopf, MD, MSc[a,*]

KEYWORDS

- Total knee arthroplasty • Patient-reported outcome measures
- Handheld image-free robotic-assisted total knee arthroplasty • Body mass index • Osteoarthritis

KEY POINTS

- Handheld image-free robotic assistance can achieve better reproducible alignment within ±3° from target alignment in total knee arthroplasty (TKA) compared to manual instrumentation.
- High implant survivorship was seen among patients who received handheld image-free robotically assisted TKA with an estimated 95.9% freedom from all-cause revisions at 2 years postoperatively.
- Favorable patient-reported outcomes were seen following TKA with a handheld image-free robot compared to conventional TKA, which may be indicative of the accurate mechanical alignment achieved.

INTRODUCTION

Total knee arthroplasty (TKA) has been widely established as an effective and reliable treatment of patients suffering from advanced degenerative osteoarthritis (OA) because it can provide pain relief, improved quality of life (QoL), and increased function.[1–4] Given the presence of factors such as significant gain in QoL, increasing obesity rates, and an aging population, the implementation of TKA is expected to increase to 935,000 procedures per year by 2030 in the United States according to recent projection models.[2,4–6] All of the above have led to efforts aimed at long term-implant survivorship and patient satisfaction following TKA.

Despite advances in implant design, enhanced rehabilitations protocols, thromboembolic

[a] Department of Orthopedic Surgery, NYU Langone Health, 301 East 17th Street, 15th Floor Suite 1518, New York, NY 10003, USA; [b] Chow Surgical LLC, 3700 North 24th Street Suite 160, Phoenix, AZ 85016, USA; [c] San Diego Orthopaedic Associates Medical Group, Inc., 4060 Fourth Avenue 7th Floor, San Diego, CA 92103, USA; [d] OrthoNeuro, 5040 Forest Drive #300, New Albany, OH 43054, USA; [e] Bronson Orthopedic Specialists, 3600 Capital Avenue Southwest # 101, Battle Creek, MI 49015, USA; [f] Orthopaedic Specialists of Scottsdale, 20401 North 73rd Street Suite 210, Scottsdale, AZ 85255, USA
[1] Equal authors.
* Corresponding author. Department of Orthopedic Surgery, NYU Langone Health, 301 East 17th Street, 15th Floor Suite 1518, New York, NY 10003.
E-mail address: schwarzk@gmail.com

prophylaxis, antibiotic prophylaxis, patient-specific implants, and computer navigation, recent studies have shown that up to 20% of patients remain dissatisfied following TKA.[7] Accurate implant positioning, balanced flexion-extension gaps, proper ligament tensioning, and preservation of the periarticular soft tissue envelope are important surgeon-controlled variables that affect functional outcomes, knee stability, and long-term implant survivorship.[8–10] Conceptually, technology that enables these technical objectives to be delivered with greater accuracy and reproducibility may help to further improve outcomes in TKA.[7] During the last decade, computer navigation and robotic-assisted TKA have gathered popularity as a tool for improving the accuracy of implant positioning, knee balance, and reducing outliers in limb alignment compared with conventional jig-based TKA.[11–15]

A disadvantage of image-guided active robotically-assisted knee arthroplasty is that some systems require preoperative computed tomography (CT) scans to enable intraoperative shape matching of the scan onto the real bony anatomy.[16] This exposes the patient to radiation and adds additional financial costs for the CT scan.[17] Handheld image-free robotically-assisted total knee arthroplasty (HI-TKA) does not require preoperative CT or MRI scans; therefore, this technique does not expose the patient to the risks of radiation or added costs of the scan.[18,19] A handheld image-free robotic sculpting system (RAS) enables the surgeon to plan the implant position in 6° of freedom preoperatively without the need for preoperative imaging. Intraoperative adjustments allow the surgeon to optimize soft tissue balancing and bony alignment by modulating the exposure or speed of the lightweight handheld burr.[20] Implant placement accuracy of this image-free approach has been demonstrated in a cadaveric study.[21,22] Nevertheless, published clinical results with emphasis on patient-reported outcome measures (PROMs) with longer follow-up times using handheld image-free RAS for TKA are scarce.[23–27]

This study sought to report the clinical results, including mechanical alignment, perioperative complications, implant survivorship, and PROMs of HI-TKA. We hypothesized that knee alignment and patient-reported outcomes would be superior to reported outcomes with manual instrumentation TKA.

METHODS

Study Design

This multicenter retrospective study included a consecutive series of patients who underwent HI-TKA (NAVIO Surgical System, Smith & Nephew, Inc.; Memphis, TN, USA) between May 2018 and March 2019. All TKA procedures were performed by 6 experienced knee surgeons, performing a minimum of 150 TKA procedures annually.

Patient Selection

Patients were excluded if they were aged younger than 18 years or had a body mass index (BMI) of 40 or greater, underlying conditions such as Paget or Charcot disease, vascular insufficiency, muscular atrophy, uncontrolled diabetes, moderate-to-severe renal insufficiency, neuromuscular disease, or an active local infection. Additionally, patients were excluded if they required a constrained or deep-dish tibial insert. Overall, a total of 122 patients were included for undergoing HI-TKA for end-stage knee OA, posttraumatic arthritis, avascular necrosis, or rheumatoid arthritis using the JOURNEY II bicruciate stabilized (BCS) or cruciate-retaining systems (Smith & Nephew, Inc.; Memphis, TN, USA). Human-subjects review by each institutions' Institutional Review Board (IRB) was obtained before this study.

Intraoperative Data

The intraoperative (RAS) registration data was recorded. The values identified intraoperatively

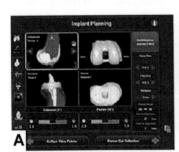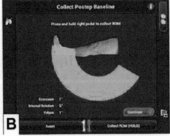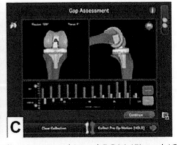

Fig. 1. Comparison of (A) intraoperative bone cuts and implants position planning to achieved ROM (B) and (C) laxity and gap balancing.

that were analyzed included the RAS registered preoperative coronal femorotibial alignment, the RAS planned postoperative coronal alignment, and the RAS registered achieved coronal alignment. These values were compared with the radiographic measures recorded for the same patients. The desired postoperative alignment was deemed as being within $0 \pm 3°$ of a neutral coronal alignment (Fig. 1).

Surgical Technique

In all procedures, a standard medial parapatellar, subvastus, or midvastus approach was used. Two percutaneous partially threaded pins were placed with the help of a pointer instrument into the proximal tibia and into the distal femur for the tracking arrays of the robotic system. Standard exposure of both the femur and tibia was carried out. The osteophytes were excised before gathering data with the robot. Mechanical and rotational axes of the limb were determined preoperatively by establishing the hip, knee, and ankle centers. The kinematic axis of the knee was identified and selected to determine the rotational position of the femoral component. The morphology of the knee was determined by mapping out the condylar anatomy by "painting" the surfaces with the probe. The systems software program created a virtual 3D model of the knee. The implant best-fit size on the virtual model is then selected by the surgeon, including the position of the implant in the coronal, sagittal, and rotational planes. Valgus and varus stress was applied during full range of motion to create tension in the medial and lateral structures for dynamic soft tissue balancing. The software creates a graphical gap space through the full range of motion by which the surgeon can adjust the desired mechanical alignment and the planned position of the femoral and tibial components to optimize the soft tissue balancing.

After planning is completed, the distal femoral bone is prepared with a high-speed 5-mm burr by continuously moving the robotic hand piece. The saw guides are then fixed, with the feedback of the robotic system. After trial components are placed, knee balance and patella tracking are checked again with valgus and varus stress during full range of motion with graphical representation of gap spacing.

Data Collection

Demographic data including sex, age, smoking status, race, body mass index (BMI; kg/m^2), length of stay (LOS; hours), and surgical time (hours) were collected for all patients from the electronic patient medical record system. LOS is described as the total number of hours in the hospital after surgery and surgical time was the time between initial skin incision and end of incision closure. Patients were followed postoperatively at a series of time points; 2 to 3 weeks, 12 weeks, 6 months 1 year, and 2 years.

Target Alignment

Weight-bearing long-leg radiographs were used preoperatively and 3 to 6 weeks postoperatively to assess coronal alignment. Radiographic assessments were performed by a fellowship-trained adult reconstruction surgeon. Coronal alignment was calculated as the difference between the femoral mechanical axis, defined by a line bisecting the center of the femoral head and the femoral intercondylar notch, and the mechanical axis of the tibia, being a line connecting the interspinous midpoint of the tibial plateau and the midpoint of the tibial plafond as described by Howell and colleagues.[28] Target alignment was decided per the surgeon's preference each case. The values for planned target and actual alignment were captured preoperatively to later compare to alignment achieved postoperatively measured on long-leg radiographs (Fig. 2). A statistical analysis of these data was conducted to calculate the difference in planned versus achieved alignment to determine whether target alignment was successful.

Statistical Analysis

All data was organized and collected using Microsoft Excel software (Microsoft Corporation, Richmond, WA, USA). Demographic and clinical baseline characteristics of study participants and PROMs were described as means with ranges and standard deviation (SD) for continuous variables and frequencies with percentages for categorical variables. PROMs included Forgotten Joint Score (FJS), QoL EQ-5D-5 L scores and Knee Society Scores (KSS). Statistical differences in continuous variables were detected using mixed models for repeated observations, an independent sample t-test, or a Wilcoxon-Rank test as appropriate. Statistical differences in categorical variables were detected using the Fisher's exact test or chi-squared ($\chi2$) tests as appropriate.

Survivorship was analyzed and presented graphically using the KM method.[29] Outcomes and survivorship data were calculated by using time of latest follow-up. A P-value of less than .05 was considered to be significant. All statistical analyses were performed using Statistical Analysis System (SAS) for Windows v9.4 or later (SAS Institute, Cary, North Carolina, USA).

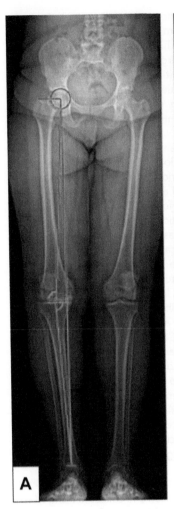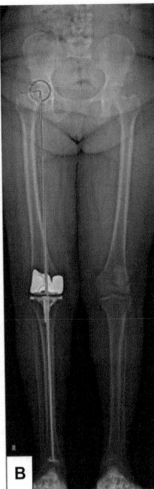

Fig. 2. Full-length standing radiographs (*A*) Preoperative showing 6° of varus deformity. (*B*) Postoperative showing 1.5° varus (patient target alignment was planned for 2°).

RESULTS

Patient Demographics and Baseline Operative Characteristics

Of the 122 patients who met inclusion criteria, the average age was 69.5 (range; 43–83) years and average BMI was 31.3 kg/m² (range; 12.6–39.8). There were 74 (60.66%) female and 48 (39.34%) male patients. The majority of the group was white (87.7%). A full breakdown of demographics can be found in Table 1.

Most patients (98.4%) underwent TKA due to a primary diagnosis of OA. The most common surgical approach used was the medial parapatellar method (77.9%). Laterality of TKA was split equally. The average time for surgery was 90.48 (range; 42–235) minutes and LOS in the hospital was 2.04 (range; 1–6) days. Primarily, patients were discharged home (95.9%). Additional operative information can be found in Table 2.

Targeted Alignment and Implant Survivorship Outcomes

Target alignment was achieved in 92.2% of TKAs (*P* < .0001) (Fig. 3).

The KM survivorship found 95.9% freedom from all-cause revision at 2 years (Fig. 4). Five

Table 1 Patient demographics (n = 122)	
Age (years, SD)	69.5 (8.7)
Gender	
Female	74 (60.7%)
Male	48 (39.3%)
Race	
White	107 (87.7%)
Black or African-American	7 (5.7%)
Other	8 (6.6%)
BMI (kg/m², SD)	31.3 (5.1)

Abbreviations: BMI, body mass index; kg/m², kilograms per meter squared; SD, standard deviation.

Table 2
Baseline operative characteristics

Primary diagnosis	
Osteoarthritis	120 (98.4%)
Posttraumatic arthritis	1 (0.8%)
Rheumatoid arthritis	1 (0.8%)
TKA laterality	
Left	61 (50%)
Right	61 (50%)
Surgical time (minutes, SD)	90.5 (29.3)
Hospital length of stay (days, SD)	2.04 (0.8)
Surgical approach	
Medial parapatellar	95 (77.9%)
Subvastus/tissue sparing	2 (1.6%)
Midvastus	25 (20.5%)
Discharge deposition	
Home	117 (95.9%)
Skilled nursing facility	4 (3.3%)
Short-term rehabilitation facility	1 (0.8%)

Abbreviations: TKA, total knee arthroplasty; SD, standard deviation.

knees (4.1%) required revision surgery during the course of the study. Two were indicated for instability (one case of coronal instability that was treated with an isolated polyethylene liner exchange and one case of flexion instability with a loose tibial component that was treated with tibial tray and a polyethylene liner revision); one case of acute prosthetic joint infection (PJI)

that was treated with debridement irrigation and liner replacement (DAIR); one case of chronic PJI that was treated with a 2-stage revision; and one case of traumatic arthrotomy that was treated with debridement and polyethylene liner exchange (Table 3). Accordingly, KM survivorship found 98.4% freedom from aseptic revisions at 2 years (Fig. 5). Survivorship analysis demonstrated a cumulative all-cause incidence of 4.32 revisions per 100 implants by 2 years postoperatively with a 95% confidence interval of 1.81 to 10.07 (Table 4).

Patient-Reported Outcomes
FJS increased throughout the postoperative time points from 11.84 preoperatively to 78.56 at 2 years postoperatively. Additionally, patients experienced significant improvement in their preoperative FJS values to their 1 month ($P = .0032$), 6 month ($P < .0001$), 1 year ($P < .0001$), and 2 year ($P < .0001$) postoperative follow-up values (Table 5).

QoL EQ-5D-5 L scores also increased throughout the postoperative time points from 73.44 preoperatively to 84.18 at 2 years postoperatively. Although there was not a significant improvement from preoperative values to their 1 month score ($P = .9505$), there were significant improvements from preoperative to 6 months ($P = .0010$), 1 year ($P < .0001$), and 2 year ($P < .0001$) postoperative scores (Table 6).

KSS were reported as 4 categories. The average expectation score was 14.21 preoperatively and decreased to 9.97 at 2 years postoperatively ($P < .0001$). The functional activities score increased from 42.13 preoperatively to 83.42 at 2 years postoperatively. Objective knee scores

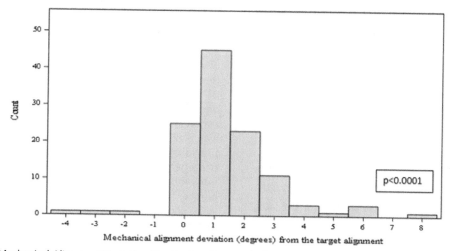

Fig. 3. Mechanical Alignment Deviation Distribution. Bar graph showing degrees deviation from target alignment for NAVIO handheld robot.

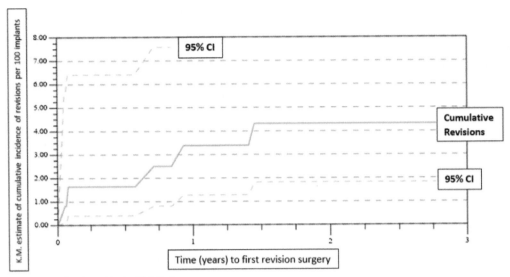

Fig. 4. Device Survivorship by KM Estimate.

similarly increased from 49.40 preoperatively to 84.51 at 2 years postoperatively ($P < .0001$). Satisfaction scores were 10.93 preoperatively and were 33.42 at 2 years postoperatively ($P < .000$). Further breakdown of the KSS scores at different time points can be found in Table 7.

DISCUSSION

Handheld image-free robotic navigation has been used by surgeons in TKA to aid in accuracy and precision of implant placement and limb alignment; however, there is a paucity in the literature regarding the outcomes in patients who undergo TKA with handheld robotic assistance.[26,30,31] This large cohort study, which followed 122 patients, who received an HI-TKA for 2 years postoperatively, found that this system achieved better reproducible alignment than previously reported, when manual instruments were used.[26] Furthermore, the handheld

Table 3
Causes of revision

Revision Causes (n = 5)	
Infection	
Delayed wound healing (DAIR)	1 (20%)
Chronic infection (2-Stage revision)	1 (20%)
Instability (liner exchange/tibial component + liner exchange)	2 (40%)
Traumatic arthrotomy (DAIR)	1 (20%)

Abbreviation: DAIR, debridement; antibiotics and implant retention.

robotic system led to high implant survivorship and was associated with higher PROMs postoperatively.

Robotic-assisted TKA has been associated with a significant reduction in positioning outliers, more reliable restoration of neutral mechanical alignment, successful target alignment achievement, and iatrogenic soft tissue injury reductions.[26,27,32] Ideally, success in achieving target alignment would limit off-axis loading, polyethylene wear, and implant loosening.[26,33,34] Alignment success in this study was defined as ±3° from the target alignment, mechanical alignment is widely accepted as a hip-knee-ankle (HKA) angle within ±3° of neutral but kinematic alignment can vary more.[35–37] In a systemic review of computer-navigated TKA performed by Zamora and colleagues, satisfactory postoperative alignment was achieved in 80% of the computer-navigated group compared with only 67% of the conventional TKA group.[38] We used an even lower performance criterion of 76% to establish superiority of the handheld image-free RAS in achieving alignment accuracy and reproducibility in TKA. Among our 122 patients, successful alignment was achieved in 92.2% TKAs, higher than that previously reported in the literature. The efficacy of targeted alignment in TKA using an image-free robotic system has been demonstrated before.[36,39] Bollars and colleagues compared limb alignment between 77 HI-TKAs and a matched control group who received TKA using a conventional technique using intramedullary rods.[26] Similarly to our study, they found only 6% of cases using the robotic system were

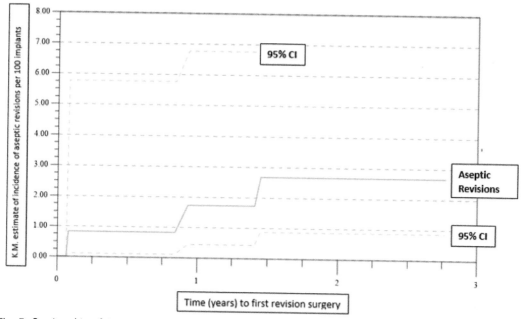

Fig. 5. Survivorship pf Aseptic Revisions by KM Estimate.

outliers with alignment greater than 3° from planned alignment.[26] Collins and colleagues found that of the 72 HI-TKAs, 93.3% were corrected to the desired alignment of ±3° of neutral.[40] Additionally, a prior study conducted by Laddha and colleagues assessing limb alignment and component placement after HI-TKA found that the outlier for overall limb alignment is on average 1.24°, well below the accepted standard of 3°.[27] Our study was in agreement of the high success rate in alignment in HI-TKA; this robotic system can be used to provide higher accuracy in implant positioning.

In addition to higher rates of accurate alignment, our study also found high implant survivorship among these patients who received HI-TKA. The KM survivorship estimated a 95.9% freedom from all-cause revision at 2 year postoperatively. Additionally, implant survivorship indicated an incidence of 4.32 revisions per 100 implants cumulatively at 2 years postoperatively. In a study conducted by Held and colleagues, outcomes up to 2 years postoperatively were compared between patients who underwent HI-TKA and patients who received conventional TKA.[41] They found a similar overall revision rate of 4.5% for the conventional group and 5.4% for the robotically-assisted group ($P = 1.000$) at 2 years postoperatively.[41] They had 2 revisions due to infection in the robotically-assisted group and one due to infection in the conventional group. The aseptic revisions in the robotically-assisted group were predominantly due to aseptic loosening and periprosthetic fractures.[41]Our aseptic revision rate was 2.46% at 2 years postoperatively, most commonly due to instability, which is superior to their aseptic revision rate of 3.6%. This may be due to the improved alignment of the prosthesis

Table 4 Implant survivorship				
Time Since Primary TKA (Years)	Number Remaining at Risk	Number of Revision Cumulative	Revision Cumulative Probability	95% Confidence Interval
0	122	0	0.00	[0.00:0.00]
1	109	4	3.40	[1.29:8.80]
2	70	5	4.32	[1.82:10.07]
3	0	5	4.32	[1.82:10.07]

Cumulative implant survivorship over 3 y.

Table 5
Forgotten joint scores

Forgotten Joint Score (Score, SD)		
Preop	11.84 (12.08)	
1 mo	17.31 (19.60)	
6 mo	51.45 (25.38)	
1 y	66.31 (26.60)	
2 y	78.56 (26.10)	
Delta Improvements (ΔFJS, SD)		
Preop to 1 mo	5.28 (19.32)	P = .0032[a]
Preop to 6 mo	39.15 (27.52)	P<.0001[a]
Preop to 1 y	54.20 (29.42)	P<.0001[a]
Preop to 2 y	66.77 (28.15)	P<.0001[a]

Abbreviation: SD, standard deviation.
[a] P<.05.

with the robotic system as alignment can lead to increased survival in TKA.[39]

PROMs are a useful way to measure the clinical benefit of this system. In a similar study conducted by Eerens and colleagues, 2-year postoperative PROMs were compared between patients undergoing HI-TKA or with conventional instruments.[42] The robotic group had an improved FJS score of 75.6 compared with the conventional group with 56.4 (P < .000). Comparably, the mean FJS score at 2 years postoperatively in our study was 78.56. Eerens and colleagues also found an insignificant higher average EQ-5D-5 L score for the robotic group (76.1) than the conventional group (74.5) at 2 years postoperatively. In our study, our patients had an even higher average EQ-5D-5 L

Table 6
Quality of Life EQ-5D-5L scores

QoL EQ-5D-5L(Scre, SD)		
Preop	73.44 (16.64)	
1 mo	75.01 (12.25)	
6 mo	78.44 (4.14)	
1 y	81.82 (5.22)	
2 y	84.18 (8.85)	
Delta Improvements (ΔEQ-5D-5 L, SD)		
Preop to 1 mo	0.41 (14.06)	P = .9505
Preop to 6 mo	4.14 (15.05)	P = .0010[a]
Preop to 1 y	81.82 (5.22)	P<.0001[a]
Preop to 2 y	84.18 (8.85)	P<.0001[a]

Abbreviation: SD, standard deviation.
[a] P<.05.

Table 7
Knee Society scores

Expectation Score (Score, SD)		
Preop	14.21 (1.63)	
1 mo	8.42 (2.82)	P<.0001[a]
6 mo	9.78 (3.39)	P<.0001[a]
1 y	9.39 (3.04)	P<.0001[a]
2 y	9.97 (2.49)	P<.0001[a]
Functional Activities Score (score, SD)		
Preop	42.13 (15.91)	
1 mo	46.55 (16.16)	P = .0586
6 mo	72.28 (15.82)	P<.0001[a]
1 y	79.35 (15.78)	P<.0001[a]
2 y	83.42 (14.93)	P<.0001[a]
Objective Knee Score (score, SD)		
Preop	49.40 (21.38)	
1 mo	63.02 (17.25)	P<.0001[a]
6 mo	78.98 (15.87)	P<.0001[a]
1 y	82.10 (14.34)	P<.0001[a]
2 y	84.51 (13.46)	P<.0001[a]
Satisfaction Score (score, SD)		
Preop	10.93 (6.31)	
1 mo	22.64 (7.03)	P<.0001[a]
6 mo	29.42 (8.36)	P<.0001[a]
1 y	32.19 (7.11)	P<.0001[a]
2 y	33.42 (5.94)	P<.0001[a]

Abbreviation: SD, standard deviation.
[a] P<.05.

score of 84.18. Smith and colleagues compared PROMs between patients who underwent an image-guided robotic TKA and patients who received conventional TKA and found an average KSS functional score at 1 year postoperatively of 80 in the robotic TKA group compared with a score of 73 in the conventional group (P = .005).[43] Although we used a handheld image-free system, we still found a similar KSS functional score of 79.35 at 1 year postoperatively. We were not able to find comparisons of the additional categories of the KSS scores in the literature. Many factors should be considered when improving QoL after TKA, including age, gender, weight, indications for surgery, and patient expectations.[44] In terms of the surgery itself, implant alignment can lead to better short-term functional results because an even distribution of the load on the new joint line may lead to better outcomes.[45] As previously mentioned, good mechanical alignment in TKA has been demonstrated in this study using the Smith & Nephew handheld image-free robotics system and may have led to the high PROMs seen.

The main limitation of this study is that this is single cohort study with no control group of patients who received a conventional TKA without a robotic system to compare patient-reported outcomes. We tried to overcome this by comparing our outcomes to previously reported values in the literature and similar studies. Importantly, our cohort demographics and clinical findings are similar to the matched cohort findings previously reported by Bollars and colleagues.[26] Additionally, the prospective nature of this study and high patient compliance in participation helps limit bias. However, due to the lack of a control group we cannot say with certainty that HI-TKA is a superior method. Another limitation is that this study only consisted of 6 orthopedic surgeons with varying levels of experience in the use of this tool, which may have affected characteristics such as surgical time. Additional long-term follow-up of HI-TKA may be indicated to further characterize long-term PROMs and extended implant longevity.

SUMMARY

HI-TKA achieved high alignment accuracy, low revision rates, and favorable PROMs at 2-year postoperative follow-up. The benefits of this system must be further explored with longer term follow-up and comparison to conventional TKA.

CLINICS CARE POINTS

- Handheld image-free robotics TKA achieved high target alignment accuracy
- Handheld image-free robotics confers with low revision rates and high implant survivorship at 2 years
- Handheld image-free robotics allow favorable patient-reported outcomes

FUNDING

Smith & Nephew, Inc.Grant ID: NCT03317834.

ACKNOWLEDGMENTS

The authors would like to sincerely thank Sherry Booz, NP from Orthopedic Specialists of Scottsdale and Ivelisse Rodriguez Pagan and Ariel Aponte from NYU Langone Health for their dedication and continued support of this research.

REFERENCES

1. Varacallo M, Luo D. Total hip arthroplasty techniques. Treasure Island (FL): StatPearls Publishing; 2021.
2. Nguyen LCL, Lehil MS, Bozic KJ. Trends in Total Knee Arthroplasty Implant Utilization. J Arthroplasty 2015; 30(5):739–42.
3. Santaguida PL, Hawker GA, Hudak PL, et al. Patient characteristics affecting the prognosis of total hip and knee joint arthroplasty: A systematic review. Can J Surg 2008;51(6).
4. Klug A, Gramlich Y, Rudert M, et al. The projected volume of primary and revision total knee arthroplasty will place an immense burden on future health care systems over the next 30 years. Knee Surg Sports Traumatol Arthrosc 2021;29(10). https://doi.org/10.1007/s00167-020-06154-7.
5. Singh JA, Yu S, Chen L, et al. Rates of total joint replacement in the United States: Future projections to 2020-2040 using the national inpatient sample. J Rheumatol 2019;46(9). https://doi.org/10.3899/jrheum.170990.
6. Sloan M, Premkumar A, Sheth NP. Projected volume of primary total joint arthroplasty in the u.s., 2014 to 2030. J Bone Joint Surg - Am 2018; 100(17). https://doi.org/10.2106/JBJS.17.01617.
7. Kayani B, Konan S, Ayuob A, et al. Robotic technology in total knee arthroplasty: a systematic review. EFORT Open Rev 2019;4(10):611–7.
8. Scott CEH, Oliver WM, MacDonald D, et al. Predicting dissatisfaction following total knee arthroplasty in patients under 55 years of age. Bone Joint J 2016;98-B(12):1625–34.
9. Boonen B, Schotanus MGM, Kerens B, et al. No difference in clinical outcome between patient-matched positioning guides and conventional instrumented total knee arthroplasty two years post-operatively. Bone Joint J 2016;98-B(7): 939–44.
10. Vince K. Mid-flexion instability after total knee arthroplasty. Bone Joint J 2016;98-B(1_Supple_A): 84–8.
11. Park SE, Lee CT. Comparison of robotic-assisted and conventional manual implantation of a primary total knee arthroplasty. J Arthroplasty 2007;22(7): 1054–9.
12. Bellemans J, Vandenneucker H, Vanlauwe J. Robot-assisted Total Knee Arthroplasty. Clin Orthopaedics Relat Res 2007;464:111–6.
13. Hampp E, Chughtai M, Scholl L, et al. Robotic-arm assisted total knee arthroplasty demonstrated greater accuracy and precision to plan compared

with manual techniques. J Knee Surg 2019;32(03): 239–50. https://doi.org/10.1055/s-0038-1641729.

14. Mooney JA, Bala A, Denduluri SK, et al. Use of navigation-enhanced instrumentation to mitigate surgical outliers during total knee arthroplasty. Orthopedics 2020;44(1). https://doi.org/10.3928/01477447-20201012-01.

15. Dalton DM, Burke TP, Kelly EG, et al. Quantitative analysis of technological innovation in knee arthroplasty. using patent and publication metrics to identify developments and trends. J Arthroplasty 2016;31(6). https://doi.org/10.1016/j.arth.2015.12.031.

16. Siddiqi A, Horan T, Molloy RM, et al. A clinical review of robotic navigation in total knee arthroplasty: historical systems to modern design. EFORT Open Rev 2021;6(4):252–69.

17. Kayani B, Haddad FS. Robotic total knee arthroplasty. Bone Joint Res 2019;8(10):438–42.

18. Wu M, Charalambous L, Penrose C, et al. Imageless Robotic Knee Arthroplasty. Oper Tech Orthopaedics 2021;31(4):100906.

19. Han S, Rodriguez-Quintana D, Freedhand AM, et al. Contemporary Robotic Systems in Total Knee Arthroplasty. Orthop Clin North America 2021;52(2):83–92.

20. Leelasestaporn C, Tarnpichprasert T, Arirachakaran A, et al. Comparison of 1-year outcomes between MAKO versus NAVIO robot-assisted medial UKA: non-randomized, prospective, comparative study. Knee Surg Relat Res 2020;32(1):13.

21. Battenberg AK, Netravali NA, Lonner JH. A novel handheld robotic-assisted system for unicompartmental knee arthroplasty: surgical technique and early survivorship. J Robotic Surg 2020;14(1). https://doi.org/10.1007/s11701-018-00907-w.

22. Lonner JH, John TK, Conditt MA. Robotic Arm-assisted UKA Improves Tibial Component Alignment: A Pilot Study. Clin Orthopaedics Relat Res 2010;468(1):141–6.

23. Shah SM. After 25 years of computer-navigated total knee arthroplasty, where do we stand today? Arthroplasty 2021. https://doi.org/10.1186/s42836-021-00100-9.

24. Jaramaz B, Mitra R, Nikou C, et al. Technique and accuracy assessment of a novel image-free hand-held robot for knee arthroplasty in Bi-cruciate retaining total knee replacement, 2, 2018.

25. Casper M, Mitra R, Khare R, et al. Accuracy assessment of a novel image-free handheld robot for Total Knee Arthroplasty in a cadaveric study. Computer Assisted Surg 2018;23(1). https://doi.org/10.1080/24699322.2018.1519038.

26. Bollars P, Boeckxstaens A, Mievis J, et al. Preliminary experience with an image-free handheld robot for total knee arthroplasty: 77 cases compared with a matched control group. Eur J Orthopaedic Surg Traumatol 2020;30(4). https://doi.org/10.1007/s00590-020-02624-3.

27. Laddha M, Gaurav S. Assessment of limb alignment and component placement after all burr robotic-assisted TKA. Indian J Orthopaedics 2021;55(S1):69–75.

28. Howell SM, Kuznik K, Hull ML, et al. Longitudinal shapes of the tibia and femur are unrelated and variable. Clin Orthopaedics Relat Res 2010;468(4):1142–8.

29. Kaplan EL, Meier P. Nonparametric Estimation from Incomplete Observations. J Am Stat Assoc 1958;53(282). https://doi.org/10.1080/01621459.1958.10501452.

30. Jones CW, Jerabek SA. Current role of computer navigation in total knee arthroplasty. J Arthroplasty 2018;33(7):1989–93.

31. Clement ND, Al-Zibari M, Afzal I, et al. A systematic review of imageless hand-held robotic-assisted knee arthroplasty: learning curve, accuracy, functional outcome and survivorship. EFORT Open Rev 2020;5(5):319–26.

32. Savov P, Tuecking L-R, Windhagen H, et al. Imageless robotic handpiece-assisted total knee arthroplasty: a learning curve analysis of surgical time and alignment accuracy. Arch Orthopaedic Trauma Surg 2021;141(12):2119–28.

33. Rivière C, Iranpour F, Auvinet E, et al. Alignment options for total knee arthroplasty: A systematic review. Orthopaedics Traumatol Surg Res 2017;103(7):1047–56.

34. Gordon AC, Conditt MA, Verstraete MA. Achieving a Balanced Knee in Robotic TKA. Sensors 2021;21(2):535.

35. Roussot MA, Vles GF, Oussedik S. Clinical outcomes of kinematic alignment versus mechanical alignment in total knee arthroplasty: a systematic review. EFORT Open Rev 2020;5(8):486–97.

36. Parratte S, Pagnano MW, Trousdale RT, et al. Effect of Postoperative Mechanical Axis Alignment on the Fifteen-Year Survival of Modern, Cemented Total Knee Replacements. J Bone Joint Surgery-American 2010;92(12):2143–9.

37. Barrett WP, Mason JB, Moskal JT, et al. Comparison of radiographic alignment of imageless computer-assisted surgery vs conventional instrumentation in primary total knee arthroplasty. J Arthroplasty 2011;26(8):1273–84. e1.

38. Zamora LA, Humphreys KJ, Watt AM, et al. Systematic review of computer-navigated total knee arthroplasty. ANZ J Surg 2013;83(1–2):22–30.

39. Mason JB, Fehring TK, Estok R, et al. Meta-Analysis of Alignment Outcomes in Computer-Assisted Total Knee Arthroplasty Surgery. J Arthroplasty 2007;22(8):1097–106.

40. Collins K, Agius PA, Fraval A, et al. Initial experience with the navio robotic-assisted total knee

replacement—coronal alignment accuracy and the learning curve. J Knee Surg 2021. https://doi.org/10.1055/s-0040-1722693.

41. Held MB, Gazgalis A, Neuwirth AL, et al. Imageless robotic-assisted total knee arthroplasty leads to similar 24-month WOMAC scores as compared to conventional total knee arthroplasty: a retrospective cohort study. Knee Surg Sports Traumatol Arthrosc 2021. https://doi.org/10.1007/s00167-021-06599-4.

42. Eerens W, Bollars P, Henckes M-E, et al. Improved joint awareness two years after total knee arthroplasty with a handheld image-free robotic system. Acta Orthopaedica Belgica 2022;88(1):47–52.

43. Smith AF, Eccles CJ, Bhimani SJ, et al. Improved Patient Satisfaction following Robotic-Assisted Total Knee Arthroplasty. J Knee Surg 2021;34(07):730–8.

44. Canovas F, Dagneaux L. Quality of life after total knee arthroplasty. Orthopaedics Traumatol Surg Res 2018;104(1):S41–6.

45. Schiraldi M, Bonzanini G, Chirillo D, et al. Mechanical and kinematic alignment in total knee arthroplasty. Ann Translational Med 2016;4(7):130.

Robotic-Assisted Total Knee Arthroplasty is Safe in the Ambulatory Surgery Center Setting

Travis Eason, MD, William Mihalko, MD, Patrick C. Toy, MD*

KEYWORDS

- Robotic TKA • Ambulatory surgery center • Outpatient total knee arthroplasty
- ROSA knee system • Outcomes

KEY POINTS

- Robotic-assisted total knee arthroplasty may be safely performed in the ambulatory surgery center setting.

LEVEL OF EVIDENCE: III

Background

Total knee arthroplasty (TKA) is one of the most performed procedures in the United States. With TKA removed from the Medicare-designated inpatient-only list, there has been an increasing trend toward outpatient TKA in ambulatory surgery centers (ASCs), with acceptable safety profiles.[1–3] Robotic assistance in TKA has been increasing in popularity as well, with the releases of multiple robotic platforms over the past decade. Many of these platforms have shown improved implant alignment as well as short-term patient-reported outcomes and patient satisfaction compared with conventional instrumentation[4–10]; less soft-tissue injury and lower perioperative analgesia requirements also have been reported.[7] Approximately 20% of patients receiving a TKA with conventional instrumentation report dissatisfaction,[11] but there is hope that with robotic technology, implant longevity, functional outcomes, and patient satisfaction will improve.

There are several differences in the robotic platforms available, which can be classified as active, semi-active, and passive. Active robotics can independently complete a task after appropriate input from the surgeon. Semi-active platforms allow the robot to perform a task while the surgeon has active haptic feedback to avoid deviation from the preoperative plan. Last, passive platforms are under direct control of the surgeon. Various platforms require different imaging requirements. Some systems require advanced imaging studies such as a computed tomography (CT), MRI, or specialized radiographs. Several systems are imageless and rely on accurate intraoperative anatomic landmark mapping[12,13]

The implementation of robotic platforms in the ASC has not been widely studied. There have been a couple studies on the use of robotics in unicondylar knee arthroplasty in the outpatient setting,[14,15] but few have looked at robotic-assisted TKA (RA-TKA) in the ASC. The purpose of this study was to evaluate the results of implementing RA-TKA in a free-standing ASC. We hypothesized that RA-TKA would have similar complication rates and patient-reported outcomes to conventional TKA in an outpatient setting.

This article represents original work and has not been previously published.

Funding: None.

Department of Orthopaedic Surgery and Biomedical Engineering, University of Tennessee Health Science Center-Campbell Clinic, 1211 Union Avenue, Suite 510, Memphis, TN 38104, USA

* Corresponding author. Campbell Foundation, 1211 Union Avenue, Suite 510, Memphis, TN 38104.

E-mail address: ptoy@campbellclinic.com

MATERIALS AND METHODS

Upon approval from an institutional review board, a retrospective chart review identified patients who underwent conventional outpatient primary TKA and RA-TKA at a free-standing ASC from January 1, 2020 to August 18, 2020 and August 24, 2020 to January 11, 2021, respectively, performed by the same surgeon at the same ASC. As a retrospective study, informed consent was waived. Patients undergoing revision surgery were excluded. The robotic system used in the study was the Robotic Surgical Assistant (ROSA) Knee System (Zimmer-Biomet, Warsaw, Indiana), a semi-active platform in which an imageless technique is used. After the initial establishment of the robot at the ASC, all subsequent primary TKAs were performed using the robotic system.

Patient Selection

All patients in the cohort were evaluated by the operating surgeon and had a diagnosis of knee arthritis. In each patient conservative management had failed, and patients were deemed appropriate candidates for TKA. A thorough history and physical examination was performed to evaluate patients' suitability for outpatient TKA. Patients with risk factors were cleared preoperatively by the patient's internist and/or cardiologist. Those with excessive risk factors (ie, coronary artery disease, diabetes, body mass index (BMI) greater than 40, peripheral vascular disease, chronic obstructive pulmonary disease (COPD), congestive heart failure, cirrhosis, or chronic kidney disease) did not undergo TKA in the ASC and were not included in this study. All patients underwent a preoperative workup, including review of medical records, blood work, electrocardiogram, and chest radiograph. Preoperatively, patients were evaluated by anesthesia to assess suitability for outpatient TKA at the surgery center. Patients who were good candidates for outpatient TKA, attended a "prehab" educational session with physical therapy before surgery.

Surgical Technique

All procedures were done by the same board-certified orthopedic surgeon at a single free-standing ASC. Patients received spinal anesthesia or general anesthesia when the spinal anesthesia could not be administered and an adductor canal block preoperatively. All patients received antibiotics (cephazolin and vancomycin, unless contraindicated by allergies) prior to incision. Intravenous tranexamic acid was used if not contraindicated. A nonsterile tourniquet was used, and the knee was exposed through a standard medial parapatellar approach.

Patients in the conventional TKA group underwent instrumentation with a gap-balancing technique to prepare the femur and tibia. The robotic knee system was used to aid in preparing the bone cuts and balancing the knee. Cemented femoral and tibial components were then implanted. The patella was resurfaced when bone stock allowed.

Postoperative Protocol

Postoperative protocols remained the same between the two cohorts. A multi-modal pain composed of acetaminophen, gabapentin, meloxicam, tramadol, and oxycodone regimen was used. Venous thromboembolism (VTE) prophylaxis of aspirin, 81 mg twice per day, was used for 6 weeks unless alternative anticoagulation was indicated. Patients received 3 days of oral clindamycin upon discharge.

All patients were discharged from the ASC the same day of surgery after working with physical therapy and after deemed safe for discharge. Patients participated in physical therapy for at least 6 weeks postoperatively. Patients were followed routinely with appointments at 2 weeks, 6 weeks, and 12 weeks postoperatively. The Knee Injury and Osteoarthritis Outcome Score short form (KOOS JR) and visual analog scale (VAS) score for pain were obtained at these appointments to assess patient-reported outcomes.

Statistics

Prior to this study, a power analysis was performed. For a power of 80%, α of 0.05, and β of 0.2, a 10% difference in complications or 8-point difference in KOOS JR scores would be detected for a cohort of 170 patients. Statistics were performed using SPSS software (IBM Corporation, Armonk, New York). T-tests were performed for continuous variables; Fisher exact tests and chi-squared analysis were performed for categorical variables.

RESULTS

Eighty-six patients who underwent a primary RA-TKA were identified, and 86 consecutive patients who underwent primary conventional TKA prior to implementation of the robot at the ASC were identified for comparison.

The whole cohort was composed of 96 female (55.8%) and 76 male (44.2%) patients, with a mean age of 62.3 years and an average BMI of

Table 1
Cohort demographics

	Robotic-Assisted (N = 86)	Conventional (N = 86)
Sex (%)		
Male	44 (51.2)	32 (37.2)
Female	42 (48.8)	54 (62.8)
Mean age (SD)	61.3 (7.3)	63.2 (7.3)
Mean BMI, kg/m2 (SD)	31.2 (5.9)	32.6 (6.3)
ASA score (%)		
I	10 (11.6)	9 (10.5)
II	58 (67.4)	48 (55.8)
IIIa	18 (20.9)	29 (33.7)
Laterality (%)		
Left	45 (52.3)	35 (40.7)
Right	41 (47.7)	51 (59.3)

Abbreviations: ASA, American Society of Anesthesiologists; BMI, body mass index; SD, standard deviation.

31.9 kg/m2 (Table 1). There were no statistical differences between robotic and conventional instrumentation groups regarding age ($p = 0.1$), gender ($p = 0.06$), race ($p = 0.84$), American Society of Anesthesiologists (ASA) score ($p = 0.17$), tobacco use ($p = 0.7$), or alcohol use ($p = 0.4$).

In both groups, all patients were successfully discharged on the day of surgery. No patients required an overnight stay or transfer to a hospital facility. Three patients (3.5%) in the RA-TKA group and five patients (5.8%) in the conventional TKA group had immediate postoperative complications of nausea, lightheadedness, hypertension, shortness of breath, or pain, but all patients were successfully discharged the day of surgery after treatment of their symptoms (Table 2).

A total of five patients (5.8%) in the RA-TKA group required a return trip to the operating room (OR), all for manipulation under anesthesia (MUA) for arthrofibrosis. No patient in the conventional TKA group required MUA. Two patients (2.3%) in the conventional TKA group required a return trip to the OR: one patient for superficial wound necrosis that was treated with debridement and negative pressure wound therapy, and the second patient for a patellar fracture that necessitated open reduction internal fixation. None of the patients had deep infections, deep venous thrombosis, or required readmission to the hospital within 90 days after surgery. Intraoperative complications included

a single medial epicondylar fracture in the RA-TKA group, which was fixed with a screw intraoperatively. There was only one visit to the emergency room (ER) in the 90 days after surgery in the conventional TKA group; the patient went to the ER for chest pain and was diagnosed with an anxiety attack and treated appropriately. There were no differences in total complications, delayed discharges, intraoperative complications, return visits to the OR, ER visits, or readmissions (see Table 2).

Surgical outcomes were assessed in both the RA-TKA and conventional TKA groups (Table 3). Blood loss, surgical time, total time in the OR, time in postanesthesia care unit (PACU), and total length of stay were assessed. Estimated blood loss (EBL) was similar between the two cohorts with no significant difference. Patient-reported outcomes of KOOS Jr. score and VAS were obtained at 2, 6, and 12 weeks postoperatively. There were no statistically significant differences in pain scores preoperatively, at discharge, or at the 2-, 6-, or 12-week follow-up appointments. Similarly, KOOS JR scores preoperatively, and at 2, 6, and 12 weeks showed no statistically significant differences between the two groups (see Table 3).

The surgical times were on average 4 min longer, with an average of 7 min more total OR time in the RA-TKA group compared with the conventional TKA group. These times reached statistical significance with p-values of 0.017 and 0.021, respectively. Time in PACU was slightly longer in the RA-TKA but was not statistically significant. The total length of stay was significantly longer in the RA-TKA group than the conventional group: 468 min versus 412 min ($p < 0.0001$) (see Table 3).

The cohort was separated into quartiles to compare surgical times over the length of the study. The average surgical time decreased over time in the RA-TKA group from 85 min in the first quarter of cases to 72 min in the fourth quarter, reaching statistical significance ($p = 0.003$). The average surgical time slightly decreased in the conventional TKA group from 78 to 75 min, not reaching statistical significance ($p = 0.35$) (Table 4).

DISCUSSION

This study supports our hypothesis that RA-TKA has comparable outcomes and low complication rates as conventional TKA performed in a freestanding ASC. KOOS JR and VAS pain scores preoperatively and postoperatively were similar between our two treatment groups. Outpatient

Table 2
Perioperative complications of the cohort (N = 172)

	Robot-Assisted (N = 86)	Conventional (N = 86)	P-value
Postsurgical event in PACU delaying discharge	3	5	0.720
Nausea	1	4	0.368
Pain	0	1	1.00
Hypertension	1	0	1.00
Shortness of breath	1	0	1.00
ER visits	0	1	1.00
Hospital admissions	0	0	
Intraoperative complications	1	0	1.00
Intraoperative medial epicondyle fracture	1	0	1.00
Postoperative complications	6	4	0.746
Dermabond allergy	0	1	1.00
Saphenous neuropathy	1	0	1.00
ER visits	0	1	1.00
Return trip to OR	5	2	0.44
Arthrofibrosis requiring Manipulation	5	0	0.059
Superficial wound	0	1	1.00
Patellar fracture	0	1	1.00
Deep infection	0	0	
Total complications	10	10	1.00

Abbreviations: ER, emergency room; PACU, postanesthesia care unit.

TKA has increased significantly over the past decade, with the coronavirus disease-2019 (COVID-19) pandemic acting as an additional catalyst. Many hospitals implemented outpatient total joint programs to help reduce the number of patients in the hospitals as well as potential patient exposure on the wards.[16] Studies have continued to show low complications with outpatient TKA,[3,17] and it has been shown that the removal of TKA from the Medicare inpatient-only list has not increased complications.[18] Robotic-assisted TKA also has become increasingly popular over the past decade. With appropriate patient selection, improved perioperative management, and surgical techniques, many patients are discharged home on the same day of surgery. Both groups of patients in this study were able to be discharged on the day of surgery and had similar functional outcomes. These findings are consistent with other studies evaluating RA-TKA.[19,20] Most of the literature on RA-TKA, however, is on the Mako

robotic system (Stryker Orthopaedics, Mahwah, New Jersey), with minimal literature published on ROSA Knee System. The Mako system differs from the ROSA system in that there is a requirement for a preoperative CT scan.

Robotic platforms pose some challenges for implementation. They require space in the OR, they are expensive, and they may initially increase surgical times. Several studies have discussed the cost of implementation of robotic assistance in surgery.[21,22] Robotics require large upfront and maintenance costs, and many robotic systems have additional disposable instrumentation costs. There also is the consideration of the costs for advanced imaging (ie, CT and MRI) for some systems. In the environment of cost reduction and bundled payments, many surgeons, hospitals, and surgery centers are likely hesitant to implement robotics for this reason. Despite increased costs in these areas, several studies have shown lower total 90-day cost with RA-TKA. The lower total cost was attributed

Table 3
Estimated blood loss, operative time, and patient reported outcomes

	Robot-Assisted (N = 86)	Conventional (N = 86)	P-value
EBL (mL)	106.8 ± 11.4	108.14 ± 11.8	0.87
Surgical time (min)	79 ± 3	75 ± 1	0.017
Total OR time (min)	117 ± 3	110 ± 3	0.021
Time in PACU (min)	220 ± 11	206 ± 14	0.12
Total Length of Stay (min)	468 ± 15	412 ± 15	<0.0001
Preop VAS (mm)	52.4 ± 4.4	50.5 ± 4.7	0.55
Preop KOOSJR	44.6 ± 2.8	46.9 ± 2.4	0.23
Discharge VAS (mm)	37.6 ± 4.7	32.7 ± 4.8	0.19
2-week VAS (mm)	36.7 ± 4.3	34.9 ± 3.5	0.55
2-week KOOSJR	60.1 ± 2.3	58.8 ± 2.1	0.42
6-week VAS (mm)	26.1 ± 4.3	20.9 ± 3.0	0.064
6-week KOOSJR	67.1 ± 2.5	70.1 ± 2.2	0.089
12-week VAS (mm)	18.6 ± 4.3	13.7 ± 3.0	0.11
12-week KOOSJR	72.2 ± 3.1	73.0 ± 2.6	0.72

Abbreviations: EBL, estimated blood loss; KOOSJR, Knee Injury and Osteoarthritis Outcomes Score Short Form; OR, operating room; PACU, post-anesthesia care unit; VAS, visual analog scale.

to shorter hospital stays and lower readmission rates in the RA-TKA groups.[23,24] The current study did not examine or compare costs.

A learning curve is associated with the implementation of RA-TKA, which is reflected in this study. There was a significant difference in surgical times (79 min with RA-TKA versus 75 min with conventional TKA, $p = 0.02$). The average surgical time of the first quarter of cases with robotic assistance was 85 min, which dropped

Table 4
Surgical times (min)

	RA-TKA	Conventional TKA	P-value
First quarter (N = 21)	85	78	0.06
Second quarter (N = 22)	83	76	0.06
Third quarter (N = 21)	76	70	0.1
Fourth quarter (N = 22)	72	75	0.3
Full cohort (N = 86)	79	75	0.02

Abbreviations: RA-TKA, robotic-assisted total knee arthroplasty; TKA, total knee arthroplasty.

to 83 min in the second quarter, 78 min in the third quarter, and 72 min in the last quarter of patients. The surgical times after completing 64 cases were on average faster than conventional TKA but were not significant. Our findings are consistent with previous studies concerned with the learning curve with RA-TKA. Kayani and colleagues[25] found a learning curve of only 7 cases with continued improvement in surgical times throughout 60 cases. Sodhi and colleagues[26] similarly found a significant decrease in operative times between the first 20 and final 20 cases in their cohort. All studies showed that after the initial learning curve, operative times were similar to those of conventional instrumentation techniques once proficiency in the new system was achieved.[27] With the implementation of this new technology in the ASC, it remains unclear if the learning curve is associated with patient functional outcomes or complications.

This study is not without limitations. The retrospective nature of the study has its inherent limitations, with possible bias in each cohort. This study evaluated consecutive cases from a single surgeon at a single ASC performing the same surgery. This reduces the risk of confounding factors but can only be generalizable to surgeons with similar patient selection and perioperative protocols. The study has a relatively small number of patients and short-term follow-up of RA-TKA performed in an

ASC. Many of the proposed benefits of RA-TKA, such as accuracy of component positioning, decreased soft-tissue injury, and component longevity were outside the scope of this study. Last, the COVID-19 pandemic may have influenced our study. There was a period of no elective surgery during the latter part of the conventionally instrumented TKA group. In addition, a small subset of patients in the RA-TKA contracted COVID-19 in the weeks after their surgery. None of the patients were hospitalized, but this reduced their ability to attend and participate in physical therapy and other postoperative care. Restrictions in services as well as patient hesitancy to attend sessions limited the number of therapy sessions some patients received. This change is a plausible contributing factor in the five cases (5.8%) requiring MUA in the RA-TKA group, although the increased number of cases was not statistically significant. In a separate study evaluating outpatient TKA at our same institution, there was an overall rate of arthrofibrosis of 3.0%, which was similar to the overall rate of arthrofibrosis in our study (2.9%).[3] The difference seen in this study is likely multifactorial, with contributions of circumstances surrounding the COVID-19 pandemic, potentially over-tightening knees with robotic-assistance, and standard sample error.

SUMMARY

The short-term results were comparable between RA-TKA and conventional TKA performed in the ASC. There were similar outcomes in terms of complications, re-operations, patient pain scores, and KOOS JR scores. One can conclude from our study that RA-TKA can be safely and effectively performed in a freestanding ASC. Long-term follow-up is necessary to determine implant survival and long-term patient-reported outcomes. With larger studies and longer follow-up, potential benefits and disadvantages of RA-TKA in the ASC can be further elucidated.

FINANCIAL DISCLOSURE

W. Mihalko has the following disclosures outside of this work: Aesculap/B.Braun, DOD, Myoscience Inc., NIH, Pacira Biosciences, Pacira Inc, Zimmer; P.C. Toy has the following disclosures outside of this work: Biomet, Innomed, Medtronic, Smith and Nephew. T. Eason has no disclosures. The authors report no conflicts of interest in regard to this work. Ethical Review

Institutional review board approval by the University of Tennessee Health Science Center. Informed consent was waived by the IRB.

REFERENCES

1. Xu J, Cao JY, Chaggar GS, et al. Comparison of outpatient versus inpatient total hip and knee arthroplasty: A systematic review and meta-analysis of complications. J Orthop 2020;17:38–43.
2. Darrith B, Frisch NB, Tetreault MW, et al. Inpatient versus outpatient arthroplasty: a single-surgeon, matched cohort analysis of 90-day complications. J Arthroplasty 2019;34(2):221–7.
3. Mascioli AA, Shaw ML, Boykin S, et al. Total knee arthroplasty in freestanding ambulatory surgery centers: 5-year retrospective chart review of 90-day postsurgical outcomes and health care resource utilization. J Am Acad Orthop Surg 2021. https://doi.org/10.5435/JAAOS-D-20-00934.
4. Smith AF, Eccles CJ, Bhimani SJ, et al. Improved patient satisfaction following robotic-assisted total knee arthroplasty. J Knee Surg 2021;34(7):730–8.
5. Cho KJ, Seon JK, Jang WY, et al. Robotic versus conventional primary total knee arthroplasty: clinical and radiological long-term results with a minimum follow-up of ten years. Int Orthop 2019;43(6):1345–54.
6. Kim YH, Yoon SH, Park JW. Does robotic-assisted TKA result in better outcome scores or long-term survivorship than conventional TKA? A randomized, controlled trial. Clin Orthop Relat Res 2020;478(2):266–75.
7. Sultan AA, Piuzzi N, Khlopas A, et al. Utilization of robotic-arm assisted total knee arthroplasty for soft tissue protection. Expert Rev Med Devices 2017;14(12):925–7.
8. Seidenstein A, Birmingham M, Foran J, et al. Better accuracy and reproducibility of a new robotically-assisted system for total knee arthroplasty compared with conventional instrumentation: a cadaveric study. Knee Surg Sports Traumatol Arthrosc 2021;29(3):859–66.
9. Parratte S, Price AJ, Jeys LM, et al. Accuracy of a new robotically assisted technique for total knee arthroplasty: a cadaveric study. J Arthroplasty 2019;34(11):2799–803.
10. Lonner JH, Seidenstein AD, Charters MA, et al. Improved accuracy and reproducibility of a novel CT-free robotic surgical assistant for medial unicompartmental knee arthroplasty compared with conventional instrumentation: a cadaveric study. Knee Surg Sports Traumatol Arthrosc 2021. https://doi.org/10.1007/s00167-021-06626-4.
11. Scott CE, Howie CR, MacDonald D, et al. Predicting dissatisfaction following total knee

replacement: a prospective study of 1217 patients. J Bone Joint Surg Br 2010;92(9):1253–8.

12. Siddiqi A, Mont MA, Krebs VE, et al. Not all robotic-assisted total knee arthroplasty are the same. J Am Acad Orthop Surg 2021;29(2):45–59.

13. Siddiqi A, Horan T, Molloy RM, et al. A clinical review of robotic navigation in total knee arthroplasty: historical systems to modern design. EFORT Open Rev 2021;6(4):252–69.

14. Crizer MP, Haffar A, Battenberg A, et al. Robotic assistance in unicompartmental knee arthroplasty results in superior early functional recovery and is more likely to meet patient expectations. Adv Orthop 2021;2021:4770960.

15. Sephton BM, De la Cruz N, Shearman A, et al. Achieving discharge within 24 h of robotic unicompartmental knee arthroplasty may be possible with appropriate patient selection and a multidisciplinary team approach. J Orthop 2020;19: 223–8.

16. Cherry A, Montgomery S, Brillantes J, et al. Converting hip and knee arthroplasty cases to same-day surgery due to COVID-19. Bone Jt Open 2021;2(7):545–51.

17. Lan RH, Samuel LT, Grits D, et al. Contemporary outpatient arthroplasty is safe compared with inpatient surgery: a propensity score-matched analysis of 574,375 procedures. J Bone Joint Surg Am 2021;103(7):593–600.

18. DeMik DE, Carender CN, An Q, et al. Has removal from the inpatient-only list increased complications after outpatient total knee arthroplasty? J Arthroplasty 2021;36(7):2297–301. e2291.

19. Marchand RC, Sodhi N, Anis HK, et al. One-year patient outcomes for robotic-arm-assisted versus manual total knee arthroplasty. J Knee Surg 2019; 32(11):1063–8.

20. Khlopas A, Sodhi N, Hozack WJ, et al. Patient-reported functional and satisfaction outcomes after robotic-arm-assisted total knee arthroplasty: early results of a prospective multicenter investigation. J Knee Surg 2020;33(7):685–90.

21. Cotter EJ, Wang J, Illgen RL. Comparative cost analysis of robotic-assisted and jig-based manual primary total knee arthroplasty. J Knee Surg 2020. https://doi.org/10.1055/s-0040-1713895.

22. Vermue H, Tack P, Gryson T, et al. Can robot-assisted total knee arthroplasty be a cost-effective procedure? A Markov decision analysis. Knee 2021;29:345–52.

23. Mont MA, Cool C, Gregory D, et al. Health care utilization and payer cost analysis of robotic arm assisted total knee arthroplasty at 30, 60, and 90 days. J Knee Surg 2021;34(3):328–37.

24. Cool CL, Jacofsky DJ, Seeger KA, et al. A 90-day episode-of-care cost analysis of robotic-arm assisted total knee arthroplasty. J Comp Eff Res 2019;8(5):327–36.

25. Kayani B, Konan S, Huq SS, et al. Robotic-arm assisted total knee arthroplasty has a learning curve of seven cases for integration into the surgical workflow but no learning curve effect for accuracy of implant positioning. Knee Surg Sports Traumatol Arthrosc 2019;27(4):1132–41.

26. Sodhi N, Khlopas A, Piuzzi NS, et al. The learning curve associated with robotic total knee arthroplasty. J Knee Surg 2018;31(1):17–21.

27. Coon TM. Integrating robotic technology into the operating room. Am J Orthop (Belle Mead NJ) 2009;38(2 Suppl):7–9. PMID: 19340376.

Remote Patient Monitoring Following Total Joint Arthroplasty

Maxwell Weinberg, MD[a], Jonathan R. Danoff, MD[b],
Giles R. Scuderi, MD[a,*]

KEYWORDS

- Remote patient monitoring • Telehealth • Total joint arthroplasty • Smart technology
- Wearables

KEY POINTS

- Advances in remote patient monitoring technology mean that physicians can monitor patients continuously in the community, rather than limiting care to outpatient clinic visits.
- Telemedicine and patient engagement platforms allow patients to communicate with their surgeon outside of conventional clinical settings, resulting in reduced health care costs, increased convenience for patients, and increased patient engagement in their care.
- Wearable sensors and smart devices can provide additional insight into a patient's recovery, including compliance with physical therapy and overall mobility, and relay this information to the surgeon.
- A newly designed Smart implant for total knee arthroplasty can be used to continuously and objectively measure a patient's mobility after surgery and may be able to detect any concerning changes in a patient's recovery that may require medical or surgical intervention.

INTRODUCTION

Total knee arthroplasty (TKA) and total hip arthroplasty (THA) have been recognized as some of the most successful surgeries that can help return patients to an active lifestyle. With the projected increase in primary TKA and THA procedures over the next several years, it is important to understand advanced technologies that could help manage such a rapid increase in this patient population. With the increase in technological advances over the years, remote patient monitoring (RPM) has grown across medicine with the ability to monitor and manage health conditions without the need of physically seeing a patient in a conventional clinical setting. RPM refers to the use of telecommunication with wearable and implantable technology to assess and treat patients. Various forms of RPM have long been integrated into focused areas of disease management, such as care of patients with diabetes, pacemakers, or implantable cardioverter–defibrillators. However, the adoption of these technologies among orthopedic surgeons has been slow. Since the coronavirus disease-2019 (COVID-19) pandemic, there has been a marked rise in the use of telehealth and other RPM platforms to provide essential services while minimizing risks for physicians and their patients. In orthopedic surgery, RPM includes several modalities: telehealth and patient portals for perioperative visits and collecting patient-reported functional outcomes (PROMs); wearable trackable devices to remotely monitor gait and mobility; and implantable devices that can continuously and objectively collect extremity

---

[a] Department of Orthopedic Surgery, Northwell Health Orthopedic Institute, 1001 Franklin Avenue, Suite 110, Garden City, NY 11530, USA; [b] Department of Orthopedic Surgery, Northwell Health Orthopedic Institute, 611 Northern Boulevard, Suite 200, Great Neck, NY 11021, USA
* Corresponding author.
E-mail address: Gscuderi@northwell.edu

functional data. Multiple recent papers support the use of RPM, which has been adopted by physicians and patients, resulting in similar patient satisfaction and improved cost efficiency.[1–6]

The advances in RPM mean that clinicians can monitor patient's continuously in the community rather than limiting care to outpatient clinical visits. Despite the rapid conversion to telemedicine visits in the era of COVID-19 and the need to promptly adapt to new technology, patients and providers have adopted virtual reality platforms as a necessary tool in this time and have reported satisfaction with the visits.

TELEMEDICINE AND PATIENT ENGAGEMENT PLATFORMS

Telemedicine (telehealth) uses audiovisual technological aids to help care for patients and has historically been used to provide care for patients in rural and low-resource settings. Telemedicine involves a range of technologies, including smartphones, computer tablets, mobile applications, and video conferencing, that allow health care providers to evaluate, diagnose, monitor, treat, and educate patients virtually. Within telehealth, two major classifications exist: synchronous and asynchronous. Synchronous telemedicine refers to real-time videoconferencing or telephone communication between the patient and provider, whereas asynchronous telemedicine describes the gathering and sharing of medical information for a patient or another provider at a later time. Telemedicine is also currently the fastest-growing sector of health care, and at many centers has become a key modality for perioperative delivery of care during the COVID-19 pandemic. Much of this growth is attributable to the benefits of telemedicine including shorter wait times, avoidance of travel, and fewer missed appointments. In addition, patients report better provider communication and access, better medication adherence, and overall high satisfaction scores with telemedicine clinical outcomes.[7]

Within orthopedics, despite the rapid conversion to telemedicine visits in the era of COVID-19 and the need to promptly adapt to new technology, patients and providers embraced telemedicine as a necessary tool and have reported satisfaction with the visits. Telemedicine has allowed pre- and postoperative visits to be conducted virtually, eliminating the need for patients to travel for an appointment. A study on the use of telemedicine in an arthroplasty clinic by Giunta and colleagues[8] showed that younger patients, patients with longer commute distances, and patients who had established relationships with their provider expressed higher satisfaction with telemedicine arthroplasty visits. Although >80% of patients were satisfied with their telemedicine visit, an established patient-provider relationship may be integral to the success of an arthroplasty telemedicine practice. A systematic review on the subject by Chaudhry and colleagues[9] showed no differences in patient satisfaction scores, surgeon satisfaction scores, or patient-reported outcome measures between telemedicine and in-person appointments. However, the patient time commitment was notably shorter with telehealth than with in-person assessments, both with and without accounting for travel time. Although a virtual orthopedic examination may lack the vital elements of palpation and dynamic testing, Tanaka and colleagues[10] established protocols and methods to standardize telemedicine visits to maximize the benefit and efficiency of the virtual orthopedic examination.

In addition to telemedicine, web-based patient engagement platforms and patient portals (**Box 1**) have been developed to deliver

---

Box 1
Examples of patient portals and web-based patient engagement platforms

Patient portals:

1. MyChart (Epic Systems Corporation, Madison, WI)
2. aethnaCommunicator (athenahealth, Inc., Watertown, MA)

Mobile health applications:

1. GetWellLoop (GetWellNetwork, Inc., Bethesda, MD)
2. SeamlessMD (SeamlessMD, Toronto, ON, CA)
3. MyMobility (Zimmer Biomet, Warsaw, IN)
4. Force (Force Therapeautics, New York City, NY)
5. Twistle (Twistle Inc., Seattle, WA)
6. Pattern Health (Pattern Health, Durham, NC)
7. Mobomo (Mobomo, Vienna, VA)
8. WellBe (WellBe Inc., Maddison, WI)
9. Conversa, tap cloud (TapCloud LLC, Chicago, IL)

Chatbots:

1. STREAMD (StreaMD Corp., Chicago, IL)
2. Conversa (ConversaHealth, Portland, OR)
3. Memora Health (Memora Health, San Francisco, CA)

information regarding pathophysiology, surgical planning, and the postoperative course. These digital health applications are aimed at reducing costs, increasing health care convenience for patients, and increasing patient engagement in their care through automated patient outreach.[11] Common patient engagement platforms include patient portals, mobile applications for android/iOS platforms, and messaging chatbots. They can provide patients with a range of information including laboratory results, clinic visit summaries, appointment reminders, educational materials, care videos and instructions, and electronic messaging. Engaging patients in their own care of chronic medical conditions and improving health literacy has been shown to increase patient medication compliance while decreasing costs.[12] Research within the field of total joint arthroplasty (TJA) has drawn similar conclusions with higher preoperative patient activation being associated with better functional outcomes and higher patient satisfaction postoperatively.[13] Patient activation refers to a patient's tendency to be involved in adaptive health behavior which may lead to improved satisfaction and outcomes.[14] To promote patient activation, surgeons have traditionally used preoperative education classes and nurse navigators to aid in the optimization and preparation of patients for surgery. These educational programs resulted in decreased stress and anxiety surrounding TJA, improved patient knowledge, and increased patient satisfaction. Digital technology has emerged as a useful educational and engagement tool in the perioperative period, particularly during the COVID-19 pandemic when it became essential to augment in-person care with digital care. In addition, with more patients having outpatient surgery (ie, same day or 23 h stay) and surgeons having less face-time with patients during their clinic visits, digital health applications allow more clinical exposure for the patient.

Expanding research in the field of TJA suggests that the use of patient portals and other technologies to provide patient education in the perioperative period allows care to be delivered at a lower cost,[15,16] increased patient satisfaction,[1] improved outcome scores in TKA patients,[2] improved clinical outcomes with shorter hospital stays, and lower readmissions secondary to fewer postoperative complications.[2,16,17] Some web-based patient portals for perioperative care have expanded to include online physical therapy, increasing convenience for patients while decreasing costs. A study by Holte and colleagues[12] found that portal participation in both TKA and THA cohorts was increased among patients who were younger, had a higher BMI, and were of higher socioeconomic class. In addition, a study by Knapp and colleagues[14] showed high patient engagement and compliance via the use of a digital application-based platform for patients undergoing TJA. Although the use of web-based patient engagement platforms and patient portals has led to improved outcomes and decreased costs for many patients, future research could study methods of improving utilization and access for all patient populations.

Wearable Trackable Devices

Although telemedicine addresses issues of travel and cost while potentially improving patient satisfaction, a virtual assessment of the extremity provides limited objective data for review. Furthermore, around 20% of patients are not satisfied after surgery and continue to have postoperative pain and functional limitations, with associated implications for recovery. Recently there has been a proliferation of wearable devices that can track, monitor, and analyze activity, but their use in assessing recovery after surgery has been limited. The advent of mobile and wearable (ie, Fitbit, Jawbone, and Apple Watch) communication devices, in conjunction with the internet and social media, present unique opportunities to optimize health and disease management. In particular, wearable sensors ("wearables") and mobile devices may facilitate postoperative patient monitoring, and allow the surgeon to holistically capture the status of patients after joint arthroplasty with continuous subjective and objective data.[3] These wearable devices may use commercially available technologies that can provide additional insight into the patient's recovery, including compliance with physical therapy and overall mobility (**Box 2**). In many cases, wearable

---

Box 2
External smart devices to monitor patients post-TKA

Wrist devices

1. Fitbit Blaze (Fitbit, San Francisco, CA)

2. Garmin Vivosport (Garmin, Lenexa, Kansas)

3. Apple Watch (Apple, Cupertino, CA)

Smart braces

1. Breg Flex (Breg, Carlsbad, CA)

2. DONJOY X4TM (DJO LLC, Carlsbad, CA)

3. Sensoria Smart Knee Brace (Sensoria Health, Redmond, WA)

technology located in proximity to the knee has been used to assess gait, whereas wrist-based wearable technology has been used to assess patient postoperative mobility. Within smartphones and smartwatches, accelerometers and gyroscopes can passively capture extremity data amenable to interpretation and display real-time feedback for the post-surgical patient. Several studies have assessed the feasibility and utility of using this technology on the wrist or ankle by passively tracking patient activity, such as step counts, distance walked, and caloric measures of exercise intensity.[18–20] Patterson and colleagues[21] found that decreased postoperative activity, monitored with a Fitbit (Fitbit Corp, San Francisco, CA), was associated with greater pain reduction and no change in early subjective outcomes after THA and TKA. Mehta and colleagues[5] showed that a remote monitoring program did not increase the rate of discharge to home, but did significantly decrease the rehospitalization rate in a randomized clinical trial after hip and knee arthroplasty. Furthermore, subsequent studies have examined how to optimize these technologies for monitoring such as the optimal body location of the wearable device,[22] and how frequently to sample the returned data to more accurately predict patient outcomes.[23] Others have studied how to couple these technologies with machine learning to provide increased streamlined and objective services.[24,25] With further use of these wearable devices with real-time statistical data analysis, surgeons could use insights from RPM data to trigger outpatient contact or coordinate follow-up based on concerning trends in objective patient behavior.

Beyond personal smartphone and/or smartwatch technology, RPM has been studied with knee sleeves and at-home exercise devices.[3,26] In a study by Ramkumar and colleagues,[3] post-TKA patients wore knee sleeves to measure mobility, range of motion, PROMs, opioid consumption, and home-exercise program compliance. Results indicate that the RPM system is a valid way to collect, measure, store, and transmit patient-related data, including activity levels, ROM data, and opioid use. All patients indicated that the system was engaging, citing the application's ease of use, real-time feedback during exercise, and daily notifications as motivating factors. In another study by Bolam and colleagues,[26] patients wore ankle sensors on each limb postoperatively to measure the linear accelerations and angular velocities of each limb. Results showed the successful collection of data from the ankle-worn device with the ability to

quantitatively assess postoperative function in patients' recovery after knee arthroplasty. In certain patients where discrepancies were noted between subjective PROMs and objective assessments with the ankle-worn bracelet, the authors suggested that the wearable device may be able to identify a struggling patient during post-operative recovery. Other rehabilitation devices available with remote monitoring capability include the interACTION system (University of Pittsburgh) and PortableConnect system (ROM Technologies, Brookfield, CT).[27,28] The interACTION system uses portable motion sensors placed on either side of a joint and attached with adjustable straps to collect joint orientation data using a custom mobile application. The mobile application contains 30 knee-specific home exercises for TKA rehabilitation, and a physical therapist or physician can offer remote guidance and track progress through a clinician portal. The PortableConnect system uses a stationary bicycle device for physical therapy exercises with an attached telehealth screen that allows surgeons to access a network where they can monitor their patient's progress throughout their customized rehab plan.

Regarding patient satisfaction, a recent study by Kurtz and colleagues[4] showed that THA patients were highly receptive to using smartphone and wearable technologies within their treatments. THA patients also expressed a strong willingness to have their body movement, balance, sleep, and cardiac output tracked using remote technology. Similarly, Bergmann and colleagues[29] found that many patients are willing to wear the remote monitoring device if it was small, discreet, unobtrusive, and preferably incorporated into everyday objects. Although studies regarding RPM using wearable devices highlight the ability to more completely evaluate arthroplasty patients in terms of mobility and rehabilitation compliance, patient compliance and device accuracy are limiting factors. Although there has been more interest in using wearables as a push toward value-based health care, studies with more patients are required to establish clinical significance.

IMPLANTABLE DEVICES

Although wearable devices have been gradually accepted as an efficient and effective form of RPM, drawbacks such as patient compliance and accuracy limit their usefulness. Emerging as a new tool in the field of RPM is the design of a smart implant that can continuously monitor extremity and joint function postoperatively, and relay this information to electronic medical records or patient portals.[30] Smart implants, similar to other smart devices, are capable of performing autonomous computing and can connect to other devices wirelessly for data exchange.[31] Historically, smart sensor technology has been used in orthopedic applications since the 1960s, where force, pressure, and temperature were recorded using instrumented implants. Although early smart sensors used strain gauge systems with percutaneous leads for power and communication, current systems have evolved into wireless telemetry-based systems that are powered passively.[32] Until recently, smart implants have been used exclusively as research tools and have provided critical data while characterizing the in vivo environment. They facilitate optimal implant design, characterize the healing process, and provide a better understanding of the physical environment in the musculoskeletal system.[33–35] The integration of smart implants into daily clinical practice has the potential for massive cost savings to the health care system by minimizing expensive complications, decreasing recovery times, decreasing lost work days after surgery, and reducing readmissions and revision procedures.[36] Applications for smart orthopedic implants have been identified for knee arthroplasty, hip arthroplasty, spine fusion, and fracture fixation. Smart orthopedic implants have primarily been used to measure physical parameters, including pressure, force, strain, displacement, proximity, and temperature.[36] When used intraoperatively, the smart sensor can provide real-time analysis to allow ideal ligament and soft tissue balancing during TKA. One example is the VERASENSE TKA system (OrthoSensor Inc, Dania Beach, FL), which uses sensors in the trial polyethylene implant to measure medial and lateral compartment pressures and evaluate the kinematics of the TKA.[37] In terms of postoperative RPM, a study by Cushner and colleagues[30] assessed a novel stem with an embedded sensor in cadaveric specimens that can remotely and objectively monitor a patient's mobility after TKA. Results showed successful transmission of signals through bone and cement, with an accurate range of motion data that may be capable of detecting changes in prosthesis fixation remotely.

There is currently only one smart implant for knee arthroplasty that can be used in standard clinical practice. The Persona IQ (Zimmer Biomet, Warsaw, IN) is a TKA implant with sensors on the tibial stem that capture relevant gait metrics. The implant hardware contains an accelerometer and gyroscope that can accurately detect step count, functional knee range of motion, and several gait metrics. However, there are currently no studies that show improved clinical outcomes with a smart TKA implant. Although the technology underlying smart implants, including sensing, power transfer, energy storage, and wireless communications, has improved significantly over the last several decades, there are still major technical challenges that need to be overcome before smart implants become part of mainstream health care.[36]

Insurance and Reimbursement of Remote Patient Monitoring

With several forms of RPM available to surgeons performing TJA, there is a significant

Table 1
2022 remote patient monitoring reimbursement rates

CPT Code	What It Covers	2022 Rate
99453	Initial setup of the device, including patient education on how to use it and how to connect it with other devices.	$19
99454	Monthly remote monitoring with daily recordings. Billed each calendar month; must have a minimum of 16 days of monitoring.	$56
99457	Monitoring and treatment management, which may include dialogue/telehealth between patient or caregiver that totals at least 20 min during the calendar month.	$50
99458	Each additional 20 min of monitoring and treatment management services provided.	$41
99091	The time it takes for qualified clinical staff to gather, interpret and process monitoring data, at least 30 min every 30 days. Does not require interactive communication with patients.	$56

opportunity to monitor and manage patients after surgery with the potential for increased patient satisfaction, decreased readmissions and revision, and improved cost efficiency. In many cases, the various modalities of RPM can generate revenue through commercial insurance and Medicare reimbursement. In addition, some state Medicaid services reimburse for remote monitoring using their telehealth coverage policies. The number of commercial insurance providers who offer RPM coverage has recently increased due to the COVID-19 pandemic.[38] The five primary Medicare RPM codes are CPT codes: 99453, 99454, 99457, 99458, and 99091. RPM codes are considered evaluation and management (E/M) services and can be ordered and billed by a health care provider or non-physician provider who is eligible to bill Medicare E/M services. Most RPM services will be billed under four codes that are split into two categories: service codes and timed RPM management codes (Table 1).[39] With a thorough understanding of the codes, billing requirements, and reimbursements for RPM, surgeons can properly bill for this program and maximize revenue for their practices while practicing value-based care.

SUMMARY

RPM after TJA encompasses several modalities that can provide a more objective and comprehensive understanding of a patient's recovery throughout the postoperative period. Telehealth involves audiovisual communication to monitor and treat patients virtually with several benefits for the patient and physician. The literature suggests that telehealth services provide comparable patient satisfaction, increased cost savings, improved care access, and greater efficiency. Patient engagement platforms and patient portals provide educational and instructional content that can promote patient activation and improved functional outcomes in the perioperative period. Wearable and implantable smart devices allow continuous insight into a patient's rehab and overall mobility, and detect any concerning changes in a patient's recovery that may require medical or surgical intervention. With a dramatic increase in RPM usage since the COVID-19 pandemic, physicians may be able to maximize their practice revenue by billing with the appropriate RPM CPT codes. Future research will discover the maximum potential of these remote monitoring technologies, and work to establish access for all patients.

CLINICS CARE POINTS

- Advances in remote patient monitoring technology mean that physicians now have the ability to monitor patient's continuously, where the patient is in the community rather than limiting care to outpatient clinical visits.

- Telemedicine and patient engagement platforms now allow patients to communicate with their surgeon outside of conventional clinical settings, resulting in reduced health care costs, increased convenience for patients, and increased patient engagement in their care.

- Wearable sensors and smart devices can provide additional insight into a patient's recovery, including compliance with physical therapy and overall mobility, and relay this information to the surgeon.

- A newly designed Smart implant for total knee arthroplasty can be used to continuously and objectively measure a patient's mobility after surgery, and may be able to detect any concerning changes in a patient's recovery that may require medical or surgical intervention.

DISCLOSURE

The authors have nothing to disclose.

REFERENCES

1. Jayakumar P, Di J, Fu J, et al. A patient-focused technology-enabled program improves outcomes in primary total hip and knee replacement surgery. JBJS Open Access 2017;2:e0023.
2. Papas PV, Kim SJ, Ulcoq S, et al. The utilization of an internet-based patient portal and its impact on surgical outcomes in the total joint arthroplasty patient population. Orthop Proc 2018;100-B(Supp_12):62.
3. Ramkumar PN, Haeberle HS, Ramanathan D, et al. Remote patient monitoring using mobile health for total knee arthroplasty: Validation of a wearable and machine learning–based surveillance platform. J Arthroplasty 2019;34(10):2253–9.
4. Kurtz S.M., Higgs G.B., Chen Z., et al., Patient perceptions of wearable and smartphone technologies for remote outcome monitoring in patients who have hip osteoarthritis or arthroplasties, J Arthroplasty, 37 (7), 2022, S488-S492.
5. Mehta SJ, Hume E, Troxel AB, et al. Effect of remote monitoring on discharge to home, return

to activity, and rehospitalization after hip and knee arthroplasty. JAMA Netw Open 2020;3(12). e2028328.

6. Rosner BI, Gottlieb M, Anderson WN. Effectiveness of an automated digital remote guidance and tele-monitoring platform on costs, readmissions, and complications after hip and knee arthroplasties. J Arthroplasty 2018, 988-996;33(4).

7. Rao SS, Loeb AE, Amin RM, et al. Establishing tele-medicine in an academic total joint arthroplasty practice: Needs and opportunities highlighted by the COVID-19 pandemic. Arthroplasty Today 2020;6(3):617–22.

8. Giunta NM, Paladugu PS, Bernstein DN, et al. Tele-medicine hip and knee arthroplasty experience dur-ing COVID-19. J Arthroplasty 37 (8), 2022. S814-S818.

9. Chaudhry H, Nadeem S, Mundi R. How satisfied are patients and surgeons with telemedicine in ortho-paedic care during the COVID-19 pandemic? A sys-tematic review and meta-analysis. Clin Orthopaedics Relat Res 2020;479(1):47–56.

10. Tanaka MJ, Oh LS, Martin SD, et al. Telemedicine in the era of COVID-19. J Bone Joint Surg 2020, e57 (1-7);102(12).

11. Campbell K, Louie P, Levine B, et al. Using patient engagement platforms in the postoperative man-agement of patients. Curr Rev Musculoskelet Med 2020;13(4):479–84.

12. Holte AJ, Molloy IB, Werth PM, et al. Do patient engagement platforms in total joint arthroplasty improve patient-reported outcomes? J Arthroplasty 2021;36(12):3850–8.

13. Andrawis J, Akhavan S, Chan V, et al. Higher preop-erative patient activation associated with better patient-reported outcomes after total joint arthro-plasty. Clin Orthopaedics Relat Res 2015;473(8): 2688–97.

14. Knapp PW, Keller RA, Mabee KA, et al. Quantifying patient engagement in total joint Arthroplasty us-ing Digital Application-based technology. J Arthroplasty 2021;36(9):3108–17.

15. Maempel JF, Clement ND, Ballantyne JA, et al. Enhanced recovery programmes after total hip arthroplasty can result in reduced length of hospital stay without compromising functional outcome. Bone Joint J 2016;98-b:475.

16. Bitsaki M, Koutras G, Heep H, et al. Cost-effective mobile-based health care system for managing to-tal joint arthroplasty follow-up. Healthc Inform Res 2017;23:67.

17. Koutras C, Bitsaki M, Koutras G, et al. Socioeco-nomic impact of e-Health services in major joint replacement: a scoping review. Technol Health Care 2015;23:809.

18. Lyman S, Hidaka C, Fields K, et al. Monitoring pa-tient recovery after Tha or TKA using Mobile Tech-nology. HSS J 2020;16(S2):358–65.

19. Toogood PA, Abdel MP, Spear JA, et al. The moni-toring of activity at home after total hip arthro-plasty. Bone Joint J 2016;98-B(11):1450–4.

20. Bahadori S, Immins T, Wainwright TW. A review of wearable motion tracking systems used in rehabili-tation following hip and knee replacement. J Rehabil Assistive Tech Eng 2018;5. 205566831877181.

21. Patterson JT, Wu H-H, Chung CC, et al. Wearable activity sensors and early pain after total joint arthroplasty. Arthroplasty Today 2020;6(1):68–70.

22. Goel R, Danoff JR, Petrera M, et al. A step in the right direction: Body location determines activity tracking device accuracy in total knee and hip arthroplasty patients. J Am Acad Orthop Surg 2020, 77-85;28(2).

23. Shah RF, Zaid MB, Bendich I, et al. Optimal sam-pling frequency for wearable sensor data in Arthro-plasty Outcomes Research. A prospective observational cohort trial. J Arthroplasty 2019; 34(10):2248–52.

24. Bini SA, Shah RF, Bendich I, et al. Machine learning algorithms can use wearable sensor data to accu-rately predict six-week patient-reported outcome scores following joint replacement in a prospective trial. J Arthroplasty 2019;34(10):2242–7.

25. Jourdan T, Debs N, Frindel C. The contribution of machine learning in the validation of commercial wearable sensors for gait monitoring in patients: A systematic review. Sensors 2021;21(14):4808.

26. Bolam SM, Batinica B, Yeung TC, et al. Remote pa-tient monitoring with wearable sensors following knee arthroplasty. Sensors 2021;21(15):5143.

27. Bell KM, Onyeukwu C, Smith CN, et al. A portable system for remote rehabilitation following a total knee replacement: a pilot randomized controlled clinical study. Sensors 2020;20(21):6118.

28. ROMTech. Romtech and the PortableConnect help patients with advanced telemedicine technology. GlobeNewswire News Room. 2021. Available at: https://www.globenewswire.com/en/news-release/ 2021/11/01/2324653/0/en/ROMTech-And-The-Por-tableConnect-Help-Patients-With-Advanced-Tele-medicine-Technology.html. Accessed July 30, 2022.

29. Bergmann J, Chandaria V, McGregor A. Wearable and implantable sensors: The patient's perspective. Sensors 2012;12(12):16695–709.

30. Cushner FD, Schiller PJ, Mueller JK, et al. A cadav-eric study addressing the feasibility of remote pa-tient monitoring prosthesis for total knee arthroplasty. J Arthroplasty 2022, S350-S354;37(6).

31. Silverio-Fernández M, Renukappa S, Suresh S. What is a smart device? - a conceptualisation within the paradigm of the internet of things. Visualization Eng 2018, 1-10;6(1).

32. Ledet EH, D'Lima D, Westerhoff P, et al. Implant-able sensor technology: From Research to Clinical

Practice. J Am Acad Orthop Surg 2012;20(6):
383–92.

33. Halder A, Kutzner I, Graichen F, et al. Influence of limb alignment on mediolateral loading in total knee replacement. J Bone Joint Surg 2012;94(11): 1023–9.

34. Kutzner I, Bender A, Dymke J, et al. Mediolateral force distribution at the knee joint shifts across activities and is driven by tibiofemoral alignment. Bone Joint J 2017;99-B(6): 779–87.

35. D'Lima DD, Patil S, Steklov N, et al. Tibial forces measured in vivo after total knee arthroplasty. J Arthroplasty 2006;21(2):255–62.

36. Ledet EH, Liddle B, Kradinova K, et al. Smart implants in orthopedic surgery, improving patient outcomes: A Review. Innovation and Entrepreneurship in Health 2018;5:41–51.

37. Iyengar KP, Gowers BT, Jain VK, et al. Smart sensor implant technology in total knee arthroplasty. J Clin Orthopaedics Trauma 2021;22:101605.

38. Couey C. 4 remote patient monitoring reimbursement tips for your practice. Top Business Software Resources for Buyers - 2022 | Software Advice. 2022. Available at: https://www.softwareadvice.com/resources/remote-patient-monitoring-reimbursement/. Accessed July 24, 2022.

39. 2022 Medicare CPT code reimbursements for Remote Patient Monitoring (RPM). Signallamp Health. 2022. Available at: https://signallamphealth.com/2022-medicare-remote-patient-monitoring-cpt-codes/. Accessed July 24, 2022.

Predicting Corrosion Damage in the Human Body Using Artificial Intelligence
In Vitro Progress and Future Applications

Michael A. Kurtz, BS[a,b], Ruoyu Yang, PhD[c],
Mohan S.R. Elapolu, PhD[c], Audrey C. Wessinger[a,b],
William Nelson, MS[a,b], Kazzandra Alaniz, BS[a,b],
Rahul Rai, PhD[c], Jeremy L. Gilbert, PhD[a,b],*

KEYWORDS

- Artificial intelligence • Machine learning • Corrosion • Fretting • Pitting • Neural network
- Support vector machine • Orthopedic biomaterials • Systematic review

---

KEY POINTS

- Artificial intelligence (AI) is currently used in the clinic to improve patient outcomes.
- Although there have been some successes, AI has not yet made advances in biomaterial corrosion research.
- Few studies implement AI/machine learning to predict corrosion of orthopedic biomaterials; many studies investigate physiologically relevant corrosion damage modes in the context of marine, oil and gas, and aerospace.
- AI/machine learning models may be able to predict corrosion damage modes from both image and nonimage data, as well as multidimensional variable spaces that may provide value to the study of orthopedic biomaterials.
- Implant registries and retrieval libraries are potentially rich information sources for the application of state-of-the-art machine learning models.

INTRODUCTION
Artificial Intelligence in Orthopedics
Artificial intelligence (AI) and machine learning (ML) are increasingly used in orthopedics to assess patient risk, improve diagnostic accuracy in radiographs and predict patient outcomes.[1–5] The transition to the electronic health record following the American Recovery and Reinvestment Act in 2009 has exponentially increased the amount of digital medical data for each patient.[6–8] This data along with biological samples, retrieved devices, images, and patient-reported outcomes may be leveraged in multimodal ML models to improve clinical outcomes and decrease patient complications.[9]

The goal of AI in orthopedics is not to replace the surgeon or radiologist at the point of care; instead, it is a tool to ultimately improve the consistency and quality of treatment patients receive at a population health level. Indeed, one of the fundamental theorems in bioinformatics, the study of biomedical data to improve human health, is that a person in combination with an information resource is more effective than that same person unassisted.[10–13] In orthopedics, that information resource may include ML

---

[a] Department of Bioengineering, Clemson University, Clemson, SC, USA; [b] The Clemson University-Medical University of South Carolina Bioengineering Program, 68 President Street, Charleston, SC 29425, USA; [c] Department of Automotive Engineering, Clemson University, 4 Research Drive, Greenville, SC 29607, USA
* Corresponding author. Department of Bioengineering, Clemson University, 68 President Street, BE 325, Charleston SC, 29425.
E-mail address: jlgilbe@clemson.edu

Orthop Clin N Am 54 (2023) 169–192
https://doi.org/10.1016/j.ocl.2022.11.004

models to predict either adverse events from a patient's electronic health record or hip osteoarthritis from radiographs.[2,14,15] The current clinical applications and future implications of AI in orthopedics are well documented in the literature.[3,16–19] Some potential areas where ML or AI may find crucial new information is in their application to implant registries and retrieval programs. Researchers could use this extensive information related to implant performance in tandem with AI to investigate orthopedic outcomes. However, translational science begins outside the clinic, and a gap exists in applying AI to orthopedic implants and biomaterials at a basic science level.

To date, the application of AI to metal orthopedic biomaterials is limited, especially in the subfield of corrosion. Despite few published studies, the intersection of AI and corrosion of orthopedic biomaterials may have clinical implications. Langton and colleagues (2022) conducted AI-based work relating metallic corrosion and debris generation in total hip replacement patients with measures of soft-tissue reactions. They implement genetic phenotyping and develop an ML algorithm that may be able to predict genetically predisposed patient populations that are more reactive to the generation of metal-derived degradation products.[20] This study, for the first time, clearly establishes a genetic link to a metal hypersensitivity reaction in a subgroup of the patient population.

Permanently implanted metal devices are the standard of care for total hip and knee replacement surgeries. In vivo, many factors affect the survivorship of these metallic implants including infection, loosening, wear, and corrosion.[21–28] Passive metals, (316L stainless steel, CoCrMo, and titanium and its alloys) are among the most used in orthopedic devices due to the passive oxide film that forms on their surface.[29–31] When this 2 to 10-nm thick film is interrupted in vivo, corrosion occurs, and the resulting damage may be associated with clinical failure.

Retrieval studies in the past three decades reveal corrosion damage modes on CoCrMo and Ti-6Al-4V devices, including mechanically assisted corrosion, fretting corrosion, crevice corrosion, and pitting.[25,28,29,32,33] Developing in vitro AI models to detect, classify, and predict these damage modes, and translating these results in vivo may increase implant longevity, decrease revisions, and improve patient outcomes. Although a wealth of information exists on the application of AI to the broader corrosion literature, few basic science studies use AI to predict or classify corrosion in vivo or in vitro in the context of orthopedic biomaterials. Analyzing AI models from the aerospace, oil and gas, and marine corrosion fields may provide insight into how these models might apply to metals used in the human body. In this review, we first define AI and commonly used AI models in corrosion science. Next, we briefly introduce corrosion damage modes relevant to orthopedic biomaterials, including fretting corrosion, crevice corrosion, and pitting. We then systematically analyze how researchers use AI to predict and classify each damage mode. Finally, we discuss how these AI models may be translated from the broader corrosion literature into orthopedics to improve patient outcomes.

Artificial Intelligence Primer

Here we define fundamental AI concepts and models that will be used throughout this review. AI uses computers to model intelligent behavior with minimal human intervention.[34] The application of AI is firmly entrenched in today's widespread technological landscape and is used in various industries, including finance, manufacturing, and medicine.[35–37] AI aims to make computers think and act like humans to solve complex problems. ML is a crucial subset of AI and can automatically learn from previous data to gain knowledge from experience. ML models gradually improve their learning behavior to make predictions based on new, unseen data.[38]

Model learning

ML can broadly be categorized as supervised, unsupervised, and reinforcement learning. In supervised learning, a computer algorithm is trained on an input dataset labeled to classify data and predict outcomes. The learning algorithm can develop an inferred function that can detect the underlying relationships between the input data and output labels to make predictions about unseen observations after encountering sufficient training data. Supervised learning is implemented for object classification, semantic segmentation, and time series prediction. Within biomedicine, supervised learning can leverage existing patient data with known outcomes to aid in future predictions.

In contrast, unsupervised learning is used to train models on unlabeled data to discern underlying patterns within the dataset. These features are otherwise difficult to determine and reliably identify from human intervention alone. The unsupervised learning model can group input data based on similarity instead of predicting continuous variable output values. Unsupervised learning applications include clustering, association, and complex data dimension reduction.

Reinforcement learning is a subdomain of ML that enables an agent to learn how to take proper actions in an interactive environment to maximize cumulative rewards. The agent, also known as the decision maker, can perceive the surrounding environment through sensors and respond to achieve goals. Although most supervised and unsupervised learning algorithms focus on minimizing model loss, reinforcement learning focuses on maximizing the total reward. At the intersection of supervised and unsupervised learning is semisupervised learning, which works with a small number of input data with labeled outputs and a large number of input data without labeled outputs. Out of all the ML techniques mentioned above, supervised learning is the most widely used in orthopedics.

Model prediction, regression, and classification

We typically categorize supervised ML models depending on the type of "ground truth" they predict. Models that predict continuous numeric values or quantitative outputs are typically considered regression models, whereas those that predict a label or categorical output are considered classification. The differences between these two categories are shown in **Fig. 1**. In addition, the techniques to determine the model's success differ. Classification prediction results may be evaluated by accuracy, precision, recall, confusion matrix, etc. In regression modeling, the mean absolute error, mean square error (MSE), and root MSE are frequently used metrics to calculate the difference between the predicted and ground truth values.

Machine learning models: artificial neural networks

Artificial neural networks (ANNs), support vector machines (SVM), and decision trees (DTs) are prominent ML algorithms for classification (see **Fig. 1A**) and regression (see **Fig. 1B**) prediction in both the academic literature and in the clinic.

ANNs are supervised ML algorithms that loosely imitate the biological neural circuit. In practice, this model is a cluster of connected artificial neurons that extracts features from raw input data. A neuron of an ANN, much like a biological neuron, receives input and processes it to produce an output.[39] This artificial neuron uses a mathematical function known as the activation function to process the input. In a web of interconnected neurons, one neuron's output becomes another's input. Next, a backpropagation

algorithm is applied to train the ANNs.[40] The weights of activation functions are iteratively updated in backpropagation based on the loss function performance. **Fig. 2A** shows a typical ANN comprising input, hidden, and output layers.

An ANN with multiple hidden layers is a deep neural network (DNN). DNNs became successful following the tremendous growth in computing power and the accessibility of large amounts of data. The popularity of DNNs played a significant role in the emergence of deep learning (DL), a subdiscipline of ML.[41] Multilayer perceptron networks, convolutional neural networks (CNN), and recurrent neural networks are prominent DL algorithms used for processing data such as images, text, and audio. DL algorithms can understand complex features of massive data that are not apparent to human intuition. Computer vision, natural language processing, drug design, and bioinformatics are taking advantage of DL models for classification, regression, and cluster analysis.[42–45] In health care, DL has been used for medical image classification to assist in disease diagnosis and research.[46] A fully trained DL model on orthopedic radiographs performed on par with human experts in identifying fractures.[47]

Machine learning models: support vector machines

SVMs are a popular ML algorithm for classification problems.[48] SVMs are linear classifiers that can be applied to nonlinear datasets. They use kernel functions, mathematical formulations that convert input data into the required form, to map the nonlinear data onto a high-dimensional feature space. As illustrated in **Fig. 2B**, a hyperplane is generated within this feature space that assists in data classification. SVMs are known for their ability to generalize and escape local extrema. Due to these properties, SVMs have been applied for medical image classification, health monitoring, and disease prediction.[49–51] SVMs have also been used for several classification tasks to investigate osteoarthritis.[16] The SVM algorithm may be extended as support vector regression and support vector clustering, which are used for regression and cluster analysis, respectively.[52,53]

Machine learning models: decision trees

Many ML algorithms are considered black box models. The user has input and output details but the model's inner mechanism is unknown. In contrast, DT algorithms are intuitive, and the concepts underlying the family of algorithms are comparatively easier to understand. DTs

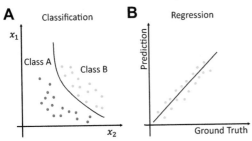

Fig. 1. The plots of (A) classification and (B) regression modeling.

are supervised ML algorithms and are widely used for data classification.[54] They break a complex decision-making process into a network of simpler decisions and have a hierarchical tree structure with nodes and branches, as illustrated in Fig. 2C. The entire dataset enters the DT at the root node, traverses through decision nodes, and ends at leaf nodes. The nodes and branches are recursively built until all the data instances in a leaf node belong to the same category. Each decision node is a function of attributes that splits the data into smaller subsets. Although DTs are predominantly used for classification, they can solve regression problems. DT algorithms are used in health care for data mining, automated diagnosis, and medical image and data classification.[55–58] Within orthopedics, DTs are used in spinal column injury cases to create homogeneous clusters of patients and study the actual effects of treatment.[59]

Machine learning models: K-means clustering
In contrast to classification algorithms that use predefined labels, clustering algorithms are unsupervised. K-means clustering is a prominent unsupervised ML algorithm for cluster analysis.[60] The algorithm starts by creating k random centroids that determine the number of clusters in the dataset. An instance of data is assigned to a cluster with the nearest centroid. Fig. 2D shows the dataset separated into three clusters. The centroids are iteratively updated with the arithmetic mean position, and the data is reassigned based on the updated centroids of clusters. K-means clustering does not require labeling of training data, guarantees convergence, and can handle big data.[61] One drawback of this algorithm is that input data representation and the random initialization of centroids influence the output. K-means clustering has been applied for knowledge discovery in health care, clustering of patient disease data, and medical image segmentation.[62–64] Previously, k-means clustering has been used to classify patient images of intertrochanteric fractures into five distinct fracture types.[65]

Corrosion in the Human Body

Corrosion occurs at the biology-device interface in vivo and is associated with clinical failure.[29] In the past three decades, retrieval studies have documented corrosion in the modular tapers of total hip replacement devices.[22–24,32,33,66–69] The use of modular taper designs in orthopedic implants began in the 1980s and has continued to be a foundational design element in total hip implants. Within the taper region of a total hip replacement, the femoral head and neck of the stem form a crevice when assembled. Both the head and stem interfaces are in close proximity and create a small volume where physiologic solution can be present. When a patient

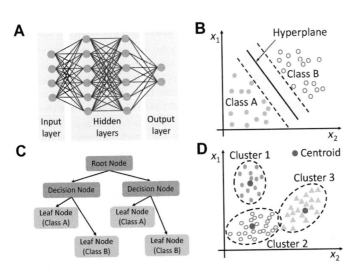

Fig. 2. (A) Structure of an ANN, (B) data classification using SVM, (C) structure of DT algorithm, and (D) cluster analysis through K-means clustering.

cyclically loads their implant (i.e., walking), asperities (high points that inevitably arise on manufactured metal surfaces) on the two interfaces may abrade the passive oxide film covering CoCrMo, Ti-alloys and stainless-steel alloys, resulting in a high rate of corrosion at the metal-solution interface until the oxide film repassivates, typically within a few milliseconds. This cyclic abrasion, when sliding distances are 100 μm or less, is defined as fretting. Fretting along with the synergistic effects of solution chemistry, pH, and cathodic activation (i.e., negative potentials that arise from oxide film disruption), is responsible for most severe corrosion documented in vivo.[25,70–74] The combined phenomenon of wear and crevice corrosion is known as mechanically assisted crevice corrosion (MACC), or tribocorrosion. It is hypothesized to promote an autocatalytic behavior, promoting further corrosion damage in vivo.[25]

In this review, we separate MACC into mechanical (i.e., fretting) and chemical damage modes (crevice corrosion and pitting). Because few research articles exist on predicting corrosion damage modes in the context of orthopedic biomaterials, we broadened our literature review to include all fields of corrosion. We investigated the following research questions: First, how are researchers using AI to predict clinically relevant corrosion damage modes in vitro? Next, how can this in vitro benchwork be translated to improve clinical outcomes?

Fretting in Vivo

Fretting corrosion damage (**Fig. 3A–D**) has been documented at modular taper junctions and acetabular interfaces in orthopedic devices. This damage can generate metallic debris that may induce adverse local tissue responses and promote periprosthetic osteolysis or soft-tissue reactions including pseudotumors, fluid cysts, and necrotic masses.[75,76] Clinical failure may arise when fretting occurs in an aqueous environment in vivo in combination with cyclic loading. On retrieved devices, fretting corrosion damage can be classified using the Goldberg score,[33] a visual assessment to quickly quantify the amount of corrosion on an orthopedic component. Devices' scores range from 1 to 4 depending on the presence and severity of wear debris, pitting, and surface discoloration. The total corroded surface area of the device may also be used to distinguish between the various Goldberg scores. The mechanisms of fretting corrosion have been extensively modeled and explored in vitro, helping to improve preclinical orthopedic device tests.[21,71,72,77–79]

Crevice Corrosion in Vivo

Although the wear damage modes associated with MACC (i.e., fretting) have been replicated in vitro, the mechanisms of crevice corrosion damage modes observed on orthopedic retrievals remain comparatively unexplored and unelucidated. Within the modular taper junctions of femoral heads and stems, the formation of thick oxide films, selective dissolution, and hydrogen embrittlement have been documented on Ti-6Al-4V interfaces.[28,32] Additionally, columnar damage, selective dissolution, and phase boundary corrosion have all been observed on CoCrMo orthopedic devices.[80]

Although tribology initially abrades the passive oxide film, promoting oxidation and redox reactions, it is hypothesized that alterations to the physiologic solution and surface potential affect the development of these damage modes in vivo. Deaeration of the crevice, cathodic activation of the surface, and the generation of oxidizers at the solution-device interface may all be necessary to reproduce crevice corrosion damage modes.[25] Indeed, studies show that the combination of cathodic activation and inflammatory species induces selective dissolution of the Ti-6Al-4V β phase in vitro.[81,82] Digital images of an orthopedic device and SEM micrographs showing various crevice corrosion damage modes can be seen in **Fig. 4A–D**.

Pitting in Vivo

Pits have been documented on retrieved CoCrMo surfaces and are found within crevice-containing regions such as modular junctions or immediately adjacent to crevice-containing regions.[29] Pitting on Ti-6Al-4V in vivo (**Fig. 5A–D**) was not considered possible until recently and has not been replicated in vitro to date.[32] Micrographs of Ti-6Al-4V femoral stems show pits 500 μm wide. When cross-sectioned, these pits reveal selective dissolution of the Ti-6Al-4V β phase. Thus in vivo pitting on Ti-6Al-4V may be promoted by crevice corrosion conditions.

METHODS

The Web of Science and Scopus databases were queried with the following topic search terms: "Fretting" and "Artificial intelligence" or "Fretting" and "Machine learning," "Crevice corrosion" and "Artificial intelligence" or "Crevice corrosion" and "Machine learning," and "Pitting corrosion" and "Artificial intelligence" or "Pitting corrosion" and "Machine learning." We selected these two databases and formed search terms to capture AI/ML articles that relate to

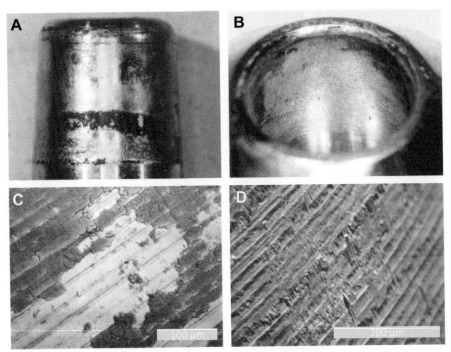

Fig. 3. Digital optical images of fretting corrosion on (*A*) exterior femoral taper and (*B*) interior femoral head surfaces; (*C*) SEM backscattered electron micrograph of femoral taper. Note the accumulation of oxide (*dark regions*) between the machined metal (*bright*) ridges; (*D*) SEM micrograph of fretting scars on the interior taper of a femoral head. (*From* Goldberg JR, Gilbert JL, Jacobs JJ, Bauer TW, Paprosky W, Leurgans S. A multicenter retrieval study of the taper interfaces of modular hip prostheses. *Clinical Orthopedics and Related Research.* 2002;401:149-161.)

physiologically relevant damage modes, even if the application in the selected works were outside the scope of orthopedics. When needed, corrosion damage modes and AI were queried both separately and together with ML to increase search rigor. For example, in Scopus, we searched (1) "Fretting" *and* "Artificial intelligence" *or* "Fretting" *and* "Machine learning," (2) "Fretting" *and* "Artificial intelligence," and (3) "Fretting" *and* "Machine learning" to capture all relevant research articles.

Research studies were excluded from the review if the title or abstract was not relevant to corrosion and AI (i.e., when querying "Fretting" *and* "Artificial intelligence," we incidentally returned research articles that described fluorescence resonance energy transfer and AI. These studies were excluded from the review). We additionally excluded non-English studies, duplicate research studies, and studies tangentially related to the corrosion damage modes we focused on. We included theses and conference proceedings that presented substantially more work when compared with similarly titled publications from the same authors. Finally, we excluded patents. We performed our search on August 26, 2022. Database searches were augmented with relevant research articles, theses, and conference proceedings that were not indexed in either Web of Science or SCOPUS. In this systematic approach, we prioritized presenting the most up-to-date research, augmenting queried articles with relevant literature. Complete details of our systematic approach can be found in Fig. 6.

Data Extraction

Three independent researchers manually extracted the following data from each research article: author, title, year published, biomaterial investigated, corrosion damage mode, in vitro versus in vivo, model learning type, prediction type, and ML models used. One additional researcher reviewed the data reported in standard data extraction tables (Tables 1–3). Attention was paid to whether the ML model used supervised or unsupervised learning and whether the output prediction was calculated through regression or classification. Various studies we analyzed referred to subclassifications of ML models. For instance, investigators labeled the neural network model they used as feed-forward or back-propagated. For homogeneity of nomenclature, we classified the ML

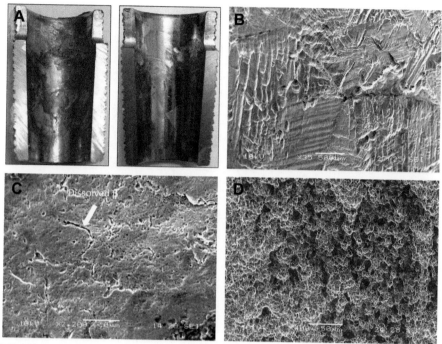

Fig. 4. (A) Ti-6Al-4V modular taper sleeve showing severe crevice corrosion; (B–D) Micrographs of crevice corrosion damage modes on Ti-6Al-4V. Note the preferential dissolution of the Ti-6Al-4V β phase in (C) and the etching in (B) and (D). Apart from selective dissolution, these damage modes have not been recapitulated in vitro. Images of the modular taper sleeve in (A) are reproduced from Rodrigues DC, Urban RM, Jacobs JJ, Gilbert JL. In vivo severe corrosion and hydrogen embrittlement of retrieved modular body titanium alloy hip-implants. *Journal of Biomedical Materials Research Part B: Applied Biomaterials: An Official Journal of The Society for Biomaterials, The Japanese Society for Biomaterials, The Australian Society for Biomaterials, and The Korean Society for Biomaterials.* 2009;88(1):206-219.

model used in each research study with the broader umbrella term, in this case, ANN.

After extracting the ML models from the "Pitting corrosion" and "Artificial intelligence" Web of Science search, 4 models across the research articles were selected to define in the introduction including neural networks, SVM, DTs, and k-means clustering.

RESULTS
Fretting
Fretting of orthopedic biomaterials
Of the three corrosion damage modes investigated in this review, fretting corrosion had the most existing AI/ML literature directly applicable to orthopedic devices. Here, we contrast two retrieval analysis studies relevant to this review that were not returned in our database queries. Milimonfared and colleagues and Codirenzi and colleagues both use AI to classify fretting damage on femoral tapers, predicting the Goldberg score associated with the documented damage.[83,84] Of the 138 stems Milimonfared and colleagues investigated, 39% were CoCr, 30% were stainless steel and 23% were titanium

or titanium alloys.[85] Tapers were imaged eight times to generate a dataset of 1104 images. After hyperparameter tuning, their SVM accurately classified the Goldberg score of the modular taper with 85% accuracy. Codirenzi and colleagues trained a neural network on images generated from 725 retrieved femoral stems. Digital optical microscopy captured four images per stem, generating a data set of 2890 unique images. Of the stems analyzed, 47% were titanium, 46% were CoCr and 7% were stainless steel. Classification accuracy of the four Goldberg scores was comparatively worse (48.21%) than the SVM approach used by Milimonfared and colleagues. However, accuracy improved to 98% when the NN was tasked with differentiating between mild (Goldberg 1 & 2) and severe (Goldberg 3 & 4) fretting corrosion categories.

Fretting artificial intelligence models
ANNs were the most popular ML model implemented to evaluate fretting (n = 10/12, 83%). SVM was the second most used model (n = 3/12). It is important here to note that it is common for AI studies to implement multiple model

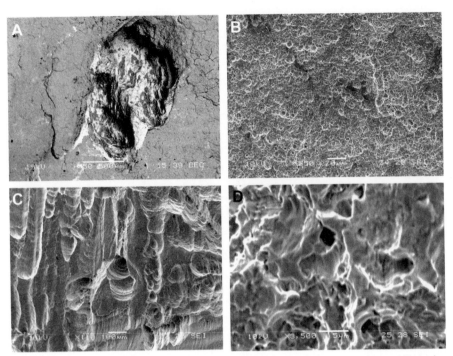

Fig. 5. (*A–D*) SEM micrographs of various pitting morphologies on retrieved Ti-6Al-4V devices. Note the variability in pit diameter. To date, the mechanism of Ti-6Al-4V pitting has not been elucidated under physiologically representative conditions. The micrograph in (*A*) is reproduced from Gilbert JL, Mali S, Urban RM, Silverton CD, Jacobs JJ. In vivo oxide-induced stress corrosion cracking of Ti-6Al-4V in a neck–stem modular taper: Emergent behavior in a new mechanism of in vivo corrosion. *Journal of Biomedical Materials Research Part B: Applied Biomaterials.* 2012;100(2):584-594.

types and compare their performance. Although only one study investigating fretting corrosion implemented this approach (using both ANN and SVM), both pitting and crevice corrosion AI studies implemented multiple ML models with increased frequency.

Of the metals investigated, 25% (3/12) included at least one metallic biomaterial. Various steel grades were used as either counter or bearing surfaces in 75% (9/12) of fretting applications. All research was conducted in vitro, although two of the studies we analyzed were revision studies involving total hip replacement devices previously in patients. Every reported AI approach involved some aspect of supervised learning. A test dataset was generated with a ground truth and used to predict either a categorical or continuous outcome. About 83% (n = 10/12) regressed a continuous output while 17% (n = 2/12) predicted classification. Fretting volume loss was a commonly reported outcome for regression models, while all classification models predicted a Goldberg score. The complete details of the extracted data can be found in Table 1.

Crevice Corrosion Artificial Intelligence Models

Queries for crevice corrosion and ML/AI returned five articles after screening and exclusion criteria were applied. Of the five studies reviewed, only one used an orthopedic biomaterial candidate (316L stainless steel). Although we have opted to include the Rosen and colleagues work in both Tables 2 and 3, because they study both pitting and crevice corrosion, we have made sure not to double-count it in our analysis or figures. All the crevice corrosion studies used supervised AI models, with 60% (n = 3/5) using regression-based models and 40% (n = 2/5) performing classification. AI models used included ANNs (n = 3/5), DTs (n = 1/5), k-nearest neighbor (KNN) (n = 1/5), and Gaussian processes (n = 1/5). All five studies were performed outside the context of orthopedic biomaterials. Predicted outcomes included the presence of crevice corrosion (n = 2/5) and various outputs related to the severity of crevice corrosion damage (material loss, corrosion rate, initiation, and propagation of crevice corrosion). Full details of extracted data may be found in Table 2.

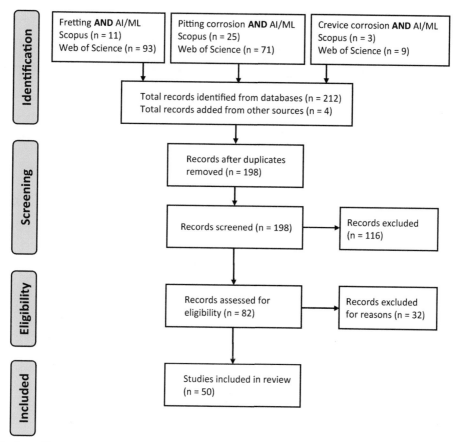

Fig. 6. Preferred Reporting Items for Systematic Reviews and Meta-Analyses (PRISMA) flow diagram showing identification, screening, and eligibility processes involved in identifying relevant AI/Corrosion research studies.

Pitting Corrosion Artificial Intelligence Models

Pitting corrosion research accounted for 68% (n = 34/50) of the studies evaluated in this review. Common topic areas included pipeline corrosion, building corrosion, marine infrastructure, and environmental degradation. About 12% (n = 4/34) of studies used a biomedical alloy, in this case 316L stainless steel. However, every pitting corrosion study we investigated was conducted outside the scope of biomedicine. Many metals studied (e.g., API 5L X52 steel) were targeted toward pipeline usage or the oil and gas industry.

Most (94%, n = 32/34) investigators implemented supervised ML models. Popular model types included ANNs (59%, n = 20/34), SVM (50%, n = 17/34), DTs (21%, n = 7/34), and K-NN (18%, n = 6/34). Two studies used unsupervised approaches, using the nonnegative matrix factorization and the k-means algorithm for clustering, respectively. About 56% of studies (n = 20/34) used classification models, whereas 44% (n = 15/34) regressed a continuous variable as their outcome. These values add to more than 100% because one study implemented both regression and classification. This ratio was much higher than in fretting AI studies, where regression accounted for almost all models implemented. About 47% (n = 16/34) of investigators applied more than one AI model in their study. Pitting potential (E_{pit}), the presence or grade of pitting on a surface, and pit depth were all common model predictions. Complete details of the extracted data relating to pitting corrosion may be found in Table 3. The number of studies examining each corrosion damage mode and a breakdown of common AI models implemented per corrosion damage mode can be seen in Fig. 7A, B.

DISCUSSION

Of the 50 articles we systematically reviewed, seven involved orthopedic biomaterials. This comparative lack of studies related to

Table 1
Extracted data from fretting corrosion articles

Author	Title	Material Investigated	Corrosion Damage Mode	Experiment Mode (in vitro vs in vivo)	Supervised or Unsupervised Learning?	Regression or Classification?	ML Approach	Predicted Outcome
Buck et al,[100] 2017	Evaluation of machine learning tools for inspection of steam generator tube structures using pulsed eddy current	Alloy-800 (iron nickel chromium alloy)	Fretting	In vitro	Supervised	Regression	SVM, ANN	Support structure hole size, tube off-centering in 2 dimensions (1 dimension containing variable fret depth), and fret depth
Codirenzi,[83] 2022	Large-scale analysis and automated detection of trunnion corrosion on hip arthroplasty devices	CoCr, stainless steel, titanium	Fretting	Explant analysis	Supervised	Classification	ANN	Corrosion severity using the Goldberg score
Gorji,[101] 2022	Machine learning predicts fretting and fatigue key mechanical properties	C-Mn steel	Fretting	In vitro	Supervised	Regression	ANN	Crack lengths and corresponding stress intensity factors under partial slip conditions resulting in crack arrest
Haviez et al,[102] 2015	Semiphysical neural network model for fretting wear estimation	Two chromium-molybdenum stainless steels: one carburized stainless steel and one stainless steel with mass quenching	Fretting	In vitro	Supervised	Regression	ANN	Wear volume

Kolodziejczyk et al,[103] 2010	Artificial intelligence as efficient technique for ball bearing fretting wear damage predication	Chromium steel	Fretting	In vitro	Supervised	Regression	ANN	Wear volume
Anand Kumar et al,[104] 2013	Prediction of fretting wear behavior of surface mechanical attrition treated Ti-6Al-4V using ANN	Treated and untreated Ti-6Al-4V, alumina and steel counter bodies	Fretting	In vitro	Supervised	Regression	ANN	Tangential force coefficient, fretting wear volume, and wear rate
Milimonfared,[85] 2019	Development and implementation of an AI system for assessing corrosion damage at stem taper of hip replacement implants: A retrieval study	CoCr, stainless steel, titanium	Fretting	Explant analysis	Supervised	Classification	SVM	Corrosion damage rate in correspondence with Goldberg scoring
Nowell,[105] 2020	A machine learning approach to the prediction of fretting fatigue life	Al 4%Cu alloy	Fretting	In vitro	Supervised	Regression	ANN	Total fretting fatigue life

(continued on next page)

Table 1
(continued)

Author	Title	Material Investigated	Corrosion Damage Mode	Experiment Mode (in vitro vs in vivo)	Supervised or Unsupervised Learning?	Regression or Classification?	ML Approach	Predicted Outcome
Ozarde et al,[106] 2021	Optimization of diesel engine's liner geometry to reduce head gasket's fretting damage	Steel	Fretting	In vitro	Supervised	Regression	ANN	Ruiz parameters for fretting fatigue damage
Qureshi,[107] 2016	Prediction of fretting wear in aero-engine spline couplings made of 42CrMo4	42CrMo4	Fretting	In vitro	Supervised	Regression	ANN	Fretting wear
Sharma,[108] 2011	Studies for wear property correlation for carbon fabric-reinforced PES composites	PES composites 52,100 steel ball	Fretting	In vitro	Supervised	Regression	ANN	Wear rate and coefficient of friction
Zhang,[109] 2018	Predicting running-in wear volume with an SVMR-based model under a small amount of training samples	1050 steel (pin) 52100 steel (disc)	Wear (Pin on disk model)	In vitro	Supervised	Regression	SVM	Wear volume

Table 2
Extracted data from crevice corrosion articles

Author	Title	Material Investigated	Corrosion Damage Mode	Experiment Mode (in vitro vs in vivo)	Supervised or Unsupervised Learning?	Regression or Classification?	ML Approach	Predicted Outcome
Bansal et al,[110] 2022	Physics-informed machine learning assisted uncertainty quantification for the corrosion of dissimilar material joints	Fe-Al Joints	Galvanic, Crevice Corrosion	In vitro	Supervised	Regression	Gaussian process model with probabilistic confidence-based adaptive sampling	Material loss
Kamrunnahar,[111] 2011	Prediction of corrosion behavior of Alloy 22 using neural network as a data mining tool	Alloy 22 (Ni −22Cr −14Mo -3W)	General and crevice corrosion	In vitro	Supervised	Regression	ANN	Corrosion rate, crevice repassivation potential, impedance values
Morizet et al,[96] 2016	Classification of acoustic emission signals using wavelets and Random Forests: Application to localized corrosion	304 L stainless steel	Crevice corrosion	In vitro	Supervised	Classification	Decision trees, KNN	Crevice corrosion or no corrosion classes
Rosen,[97] 1992	Corrosion prediction from polarization scans using an ANN integrated with an expert system	Hastelloy C-276, 316 stainless steel,	Pitting, Crevice Corrosion, General Corrosion	In vitro	Supervised	Classification	ANN	Presence of pitting corrosion, crevice corrosion, and whether general corrosion should be considered
Trasatti,[112] 1996	Crevice corrosion: a neural network approach	Various stainless steels	Crevice corrosion	In vitro	Supervised	Classification	ANN	Initiation and propagation of crevice corrosion

Table 3
Extracted data from pitting corrosion articles

Author	Title	Material Investigated	Corrosion Damage Mode	Experiment Mode (in vitro vs in vivo)	Supervised or Unsupervised Learning?	Regression or Classification?	ML Approach	Predicted Outcome
Agrawa,[113] 2022	The use of machine learning and metaheuristic algorithm for wear performance optimization of AISI 1040 steel and investigation of corrosion resistance	AISI 1040 Steel	Wear, Pitting	In vitro	Supervised	Regression	ANN	Process parameters, wear rate
Ahuja,[114] 2021	Optimized deep learning framework for detecting pitting corrosion based on image segmentation		Pitting	In vitro	Supervised	Classification		
Ampazis,[115] 2010	Prediction of Aircraft Aluminum Alloys Tensile Mechanical Properties Degradation Using Support Vector Machines	Al 2024-T3 Aluminum Alloy	Pitting	In vitro	Supervised	Regression	SVM	Yield strength, tensile strength, elongation to fracture, strain energy density
Ben Seghier et al,[116] 2021	Advanced intelligence frameworks for predicting maximum pitting corrosion depth in oil and gas pipelines	Not specified, metallic pipelines	Pitting	In vitro	Supervised	Regression	ANN, Decision Tree, Multivariate Adaptive Regression Splines, Locally Weighted Polynomials, Kriging, Extreme Learning Machines	Maximum pitting corrosion depth
Boucherit et al,[117] 2021	Pitting corrosion prediction from cathodic data: application of machine learning	Carbon Steel	Pitting	In vitro	Supervised	Regression	ANN	Pitting potential
Boucherit et al,[118] 2019	Modeling input data interactions for the optimization of ANNs used in the prediction of pitting corrosion	0.2% Carbon Steel	Pitting	In vitro	Supervised	Regression	ANN	Pitting potential
Boukhar et al,[119] 2018	Optimization of learning algorithms in the prediction of pitting corrosion	0.18% Carbon Steel	Pitting	In vitro	Supervised	Regression	ANN, SVM, K-NN, Decision Tree	Pitting potential
Boukhar et al,[120] 2017	Artificial Intelligence to Predict Inhibition Performance of Pitting Corrosion	0.18% Carbon Steel	Pitting	In vitro	Supervised	Regression	ANN, SVM, K-NN, Decision Tree, KBP, LDA, Adaptive neuro-fuzzy inference systems	Pitting potential
Chou,[121] 2017	The use of AI combiners for modeling steel pitting risk and corrosion rate	Steel Rebar, 3C Steel	Pitting	In vitro	Supervised	Regression	ANN, SVM, Decision Tree, Linear Regression	Pitting corrosion risk, corrosion rate
Enikeev et al,[122] 2018	Machine learning in the problem of recognition of pitting corrosion on aluminum surfaces	Aluminum	Pitting	In vitro	Supervised	Classification	SVM	Hydrogen bubble detection
Hoang et al,[123] 2020	Image processing-based pitting corros on detection using metaheuristic optimized multilevel image thresholding and machine-learning approaches	Not specified	Pitting	In vitro	Supervised	Classification	SVM, Decision Trees, ANN, Linear Population Size Reduction (LSHADE)	Detection of pits in images

Reference	Title	Material	Corrosion type	Testing	Learning	Task	Algorithm	Application
Ji et al,[124] 2015	Prediction of stress concentration factor of corrosion pits on buried pipes by least squares support vector machine	Not specified, metallic pipelines	Pitting	In vitro	Supervised	Regression	SVM	Stress concentration factor
Jiménez-Come et al,[92] 2014	An automatic pitting corrosion detection approach for 316L stainless steel	316L stainless steel	Pitting	In vitro	Supervised	Classification	ANN, SVM, Decision Tree, KNN	Solution temperatures and concentrations that induce pitting corrosion
Jiménez-Come et al,[93] 2012	Pitting corrosion behavior of austenitic stainless steel using AI techniques	EN 1.4404 stainless steel	Pitting	In vitro	Supervised	Classification	Decision Trees, Discriminant Analysis, KNN, ANN, SVM	Environmental factors affecting pitting corrosion
Jiménez-Come et al,[94] 2012	Pitting Corrosion Detection of Austenitic Stainless Steel EN 1.4404 in MgCl2 solutions using a Machine Learning Approach	EN 1.4404 stainless steel	Pitting	In vitro	Supervised	Classification	Decision Trees, Discriminant Analysis, KNN, ANN	Environmental factors affecting pitting corrosion
Jiménez-Come et al,[125] 2019	A support vector machine-based ensemble algorithm for pitting corrosion modeling of EN 1.4404 stainless steel in sodium chloride solutions	EN 1.4404 stainless steel	Pitting	In vitro	Supervised	Classification	SVM	Environmental factors affecting pitting corrosion and breakdown potential modeling
Kankar et al,[126] 201	Fault diagnosis of ball bearings using machine learning methods	Ball bearings	Pitting	In vitro	Supervised	Classification	ANN, SVM	Bearing fault type
Kubisztal et al,[127] 2020	Corrosion damage of 316L steel surface examined using statistical methods and ANN	316L stainless steel	Pitting	In vitro	Supervised	Regression	ANN	Corrosion degree
Li et al,[128] 2019	Determination of Corrosion Types from Electrochemical Noise by Gradient Boosting Decision Tree Method	X65 Steel, 304 stainless steel	Passivation, uniform corrosion, pitting	In vitro	Supervised	Classification	Decision Tree	Corrosion type
Li et al,[129] 2021	A Novel Framework for Early Pitting Fault Diagnosis of Rotating Machinery Based on Dilated CNN Combined With Spatial Dropout	Not specified; gears	Pitting	In vitro	Supervised	Classification	ANN	Fault diagnosis
Liu et al,[130] 2017	On-stream inspection for pitting corrosion defect of pressure vessels for intelligent and safe manufacturing	304 stainless steel	Pitting	In vitro	Supervised	Binary Classification	Adaptive neuro-fuzzy inference systems	Presence of pitting Corrosion
Lu et al,[131] 2022	A Feature Selection-Based Intelligent Framework for Predicting Maximum Depth of Corroded Pipeline Defects	Not specified; metallic pipelines	Pitting	In vitro	Supervised	Regression	SVM, 8 benchmark models	Pitting corrosion depth
Pidaparti,[132] 2007	Neural network mapping of corrosion induced chemical elements degradation in aircraft aluminum	Aluminum 2024-T3	Pitting	In vitro	Supervised	Regression	ANN	Degradation behavior due to metal corrosion

(continued on next page)

Table 3
(continued)

Author	Title	Material Investigated	Corrosion Damage Mode	Experiment Mode (in vitro vs in vivo)	Supervised or Unsupervised Learning?	Regression or Classification?	ML Approach	Predicted Outcome
Pinto et al,[133] 2022	Nonintrusive internal corrosion characterization using the potential drop technique for electrical mapping and machine learning	AISI 304 steel	Pitting	In vitro	Supervised	Classification, regression	KNN, SVM, Decision Trees, Gradient boosting, Extreme Gradient boosting, ANN	Damage depth, damage Severity
Qu et al,[134] 2021	Pitting judgment model based on machine learning and feature optimization methods	Pipeline steels	Pitting	In vitro	Supervised	Classification	SVM, Decision Trees, Naive Bayes, Gradient boosting, KNN	Occurrence of pitting and the key factors that influence it
Rosen et al,[97] 1992	Corrosion prediction from polarization scans using an ANN with an integrated expert system	Hastelloy C-276, 316 stainless steel,	Pitting, Crevice Corrosion, General Corrosion	In vitro	Supervised	Classification	ANN	Presence of pitting corrosion, crevice corrosion, and whether general corrosion should be considered
Roy et al,[135] 2018	Effect of heterogeneities on pitting potential of line pipe steels: An adaptive neuro-fuzzy approach	Pipeline steels, API X60 steel alloys	Pitting	In vitro	Supervised	Regression	Adaptive Neuro Fuzzy Inference System	Pitting potential
Sanchez et al,[136] 2020	Corrosion grade classification: a machine learning approach	M4140 steel	Pitting, general corrosion	In vitro	Supervised	Classification	SVM, Bag-of-Features	Corrosion grade
Shin et al,[137] 2020	A study on the condition-based maintenance evaluation system of smart plant device using CNN	Not specified	Pitting	In vitro	Supervised	Classification	ANN	Pitting corrosion grade
Takara et al,[138] 2022	Analysis of the elemental effects on the surface potential of aluminum alloy using machine learning	Al-Mg-Si-Cu alloys	Pitting, selective dissolution	In vitro	Unsupervised	Classification	NMF	Compound class, matrix phase class
Urda et al,[139] 2013	A constructive neural network to predict pitting corrosion status of stainless steel	316L stainless steel	Pitting	In vitro	Supervised	Classification	ANN, LDA, KNN, SVM, Naïve Bayes	Pitting corrosion status
Wei et al,[140] 2020	Shear strength prediction of TCSWs with artificial pitting based on ANN	steel	Pitting	In vitro	Supervised	Regression	ANN	Shear strength
Yajima et al,[141] 2015	A clustering based method to evaluate soil corrosivity for pipeline external integrity management	API 5L X52 steel	Wall thickness as a proxy for pitting	In vitro	Unsupervised	Classification	k-means clustering, Gaussian mixture modeling	Soil corrosivity classes
Zhang, et al,[142] 2015	Corrosion pitting damage detection of rolling bearings using data mining techniques	Not specified; rolling bearings	Pitting	In vitro	Supervised	Classification	Support vector data descriptor, ANN, SVM	Fault diagnosis

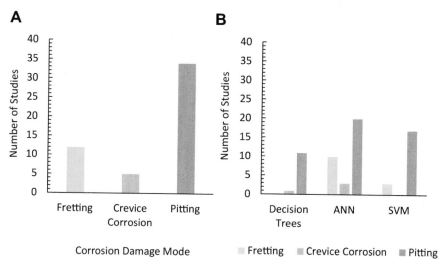

Fig. 7. (A) The number of studies investigated in the review by corrosion damage mode; (B) A breakdown of the number of articles that implement a DT, ANN, or SVM AI model by corrosion damage mode.

orthopedics may be due to several factors. First, implementation of AI models often requires interdisciplinary collaboration between subject matter experts (biomaterials, orthopedics, corrosion, and so forth) and those with domain expertise in AI/ML. However, expertise in one subject matter may not be enough to design an AI experiment, choose and implement a successful model, and disseminate that information clearly and concisely such that others can build off the study or implement the model onto a new dataset. Similarly, those with AI expertise may be far removed from the clinic, lacking the skills and knowledge to identify gaps in clinical care or target areas that AI can improve. Clinicians and basic science researchers armed with a fundamental, if high-level, overview of AI paired with data scientists who appreciate the pain points in clinical care may be able to generate and implement AI models that can make an impact in the clinic. The NSF has recognized the importance of interdisciplinary collaborations, launching funding programs targeted toward implementing AI that can improve biomedicine or public health.

Our database searches returned more pitting corrosion studies than crevice corrosion or fretting corrosion. This is mainly because pitting is one of the primary mechanisms of material loss and failure for steel pipelines.[86,87] Although corrosion failure of a medical device may or may not induce clinical failure for a single patient, corrosion failure of a pipeline can cause multiple deaths and environmental consequences, with the societal cost estimated in billions of dollars.[86–89] Additionally, access to real-world data is more readily available for oil and gas studies. Pipeline steel may be evaluated using a potentiostat, and corrosion damage can be reproduced in environments representative of the atmospheric or soil conditions the alloys interact with in real-world use. In contrast, collecting corrosion data in vivo is challenging, and recapitulating the complex factors at the device biology interface in vitro remains a gap.

Severe corrosion documented on orthopedic retrievals is associated with mechanically assisted crevice corrosion. For metals used in total hip arthroplasties, including titanium and cobalt chrome alloys, pitting is induced by a complex combination of solution chemistry, oxide structure and function, and the biology present at the metal interface.[90] Unlike steel alloys, including 316L, cobalt chrome and titanium alloy pitting cannot be reproduced in vitro by statically applying a specific breakdown or pitting potential. Many models exist for wear and tribocorrosion of titanium and cobalt chrome alloys. However, few in vitro tests exist that induce crevice corrosion damage modes, including hydrogen embrittlement, pitting, and oxide accumulation. Indeed, the US Food and Drug Administration (FDA) identified the lack of effective preclinical crevice corrosion tests as a gap in a 2019 white paper.[91] Thus, a lack of AI-crevice-corrosion experiments in the context of biomaterials may be explained by the comparatively poor ability to reproduce crevice corrosion in the laboratory under physiologically relevant conditions.

Although gaps exist in our ability to model clinically relevant corrosion damage modes outside the human body, several studies we examined in this review may provide insight into how to identify critical variable spaces for solution chemistries and potentials that more accurately model the biological milieu. Jimenez and colleagues implemented SVM and ANN models to predict the two-dimensional chloride solution concentration and temperature area that would induce pitting corrosion on 316L stainless steel.[92] Jimenez and colleagues additionally predicted a variable space that would corrode austenitic stainless steel, training their model with four variables: chloride ion concentration, pH, critical pitting potential, and temperature.[93,94]

The current paradigm for generating preclinical data and material selection for orthopedic devices is to evaluate the corrosion properties of metal samples or devices in saline solutions. Although these electrolytes may match the isotonic properties of the in vivo environment, they fail to include the array of lymphocytes, macrophages, and proteins attracted to the device once implanted. When confronted with a foreign body (i.e., the implant), lymphocytes and macrophages can promote oxidizers including hydrogen peroxide, hydroxide radicals, peroxynitrites, hypochlorous acid, and hydrochloric acid at the device interface.[90] Fretting, a common phenomenon in modular taper designs, may provide an additional source of reactive oxygen species (ROS).[95] What is currently being modeled with salt water is a multidimensional variable space and our simplification of the in vivo solution presents a challenge when trying to understand the mechanisms of crevice corrosion damage modes in vitro. AI, especially SVM and ANN models, may help elucidate the critical solution concentrations of ROS and pH necessary to induce crevice corrosion damage modes in vitro, reducing the experimental time and number of tests needed. Besides mechanistic understanding, a more representative testing solution would aid in detecting poor device designs before clinical use.

The ability of AI to classify images of corrosion damage in vitro may have the potential to influence clinical care. In this study, we reviewed two retrieval programs that implemented AI models to classify fretting corrosion on femoral tapers. We additionally reviewed various in vitro models that classified corrosion damage modes from image-based data. One retrieval study used digital optical microscopy to generate their dataset, and the second study classified digital photographs of the taper surface.[83-85] This latter approach is closer to the original application of the Goldberg score, a method intended to classify modular taper corrosion damage based on a quick visual assessment.[33] Although these orthopedic devices were removed from the patient and cleaned before imaging, the ability to classify the corrosion damage on a taper midrevision may decrease the time needed for surgery and improve clinical outcomes. Midrevision, the surgeon separates the femoral head from the femoral stem and must decide whether to replace just the head or both femoral components. Replacing the stem is an invasive process and can result in increased complications when patients have poor bone density and bone volume loss. Applying this classification model to photos of the taper would provide additional information to the surgeon, improving decision-making in the operating room.

Many studies we reviewed applied AI to classify and predict corrosion damage modes from non-image-based data. Morizet and colleagues classified crevice corrosion from acoustic emission signals.[96] Rosen and colleagues predicted various stages of pitting, general, and crevice corrosion damage on 316L stainless steel using features extracted from polarization scans.[97] Recent studies show that corrosion damage modes on retrieved orthopedic devices have unique electrochemical impedance spectroscopy (EIS) signatures.[98,99] With the miniaturization of potentiostats (pocket potentiostats) the near field, EIS method may be a way to classify corrosion damage modes in the absence of imaging, providing decision support to surgeons and researchers. However, further research is required. Future studies would need to build a dataset of near field EIS signatures on retrievals before AI implementation.

SUMMARY

In this review, we systematically evaluated the existing corrosion AI literature, looking for applications of AI/ML models on physiologically relevant corrosion damage modes. We identified several experimental designs that may be implemented on orthopedic biomaterials, including classifying pitting, fretting, and crevice corrosion damage modes from image and non-image-based data as well as predicting critical variable conditions that promote corrosion. Understanding successful models in the broader corrosion literature may aid in developing basic science studies with translational potential.

CLINICS CARE POINTS

- AI is already being used in the clinic and can improve patient outcomes.

- Although there have been some successes, there is a lack of translational studies beginning at a basic science level.

- The broader corrosion field has rapidly adopted AI models predicting corrosion damage modes relevant to orthopedics.

- Translating these models to investigate orthopedic alloys has the potential to improve preclinical device testing and provide decision support to clinicians.

- Fully delivering on the promise of AI in orthopedics may require increased collaboration and knowledge transfer between clinicians, basic science researchers, and data scientists.

DISCLOSURE

M.A. Kurtz has none; R.Yang: None; M.S.R. Elapolu: None; A.C. Wessinger: None; W. Nelson: Employee of DePuy Synthes; K. Alaniz: None; R. Rai: None; J.L. Gilbert: Research support to Clemson University: DePuy Synthes, Bayer; Consulting for: DePuy Synthes, Smith and Nephew, Omni Lifesciences, Naples Community Hospital, Stryker Inc., Bausch and Lomb; Editor-in-Chief, Journal of Biomedical Materials Research – Part B: Applied Biomaterials, a J Wiley publication; Council, Society for Biomaterials.

ACKNOWLEDGEMENTS

The authors thank Hamilton Baker, MD, for his insight and in-depth discussions while preparing this article. The authors acknowledge and thank Danieli C. Rodrigues, PhD, for her contribution of previously unpublished micrographs (captured around 2009) to this article. The authors additionally thank the Clemson-MUSC AI Hub for their help in organizing this collaboration. Finally, this study was partially supported by the Wyss endowment.

REFERENCES

1. Jamaludin A, Lootus M, Kadir T, et al. ISSLS PRIZE IN BIOENGINEERING SCIENCE 2017: automation of reading of radiological features from magnetic resonance images (MRIs) of the lumbar spine without human intervention is comparable with an expert radiologist. Eur Spine J 2017;26(5):1374–83.

2. Xue Y, Zhang R, Deng Y, et al. A preliminary examination of the diagnostic value of deep learning in hip osteoarthritis. PloS one 2017; 12(6):e0178992.

3. Han X-G, Tian W. Artificial intelligence in orthopedic surgery: current state and future perspective. Chin Med J 2019;132(21):2521–3.

4. Cabitza F, Locoro A, Banfi G. Machine learning in orthopedics: a literature review. Front Bioeng Biotechnol 2018;6:75.

5. Helm JM, Swiergosz AM, Haeberle HS, et al. Machine learning and artificial intelligence: definitions, applications, and future directions. Curr Rev Musculoskelet Med 2020;13(1):69–76.

6. White SE. A review of big data in health care: challenges and opportunities. Open access bioinformatics 2014;6:13.

7. Atherton J. Development of the electronic health record. Virtual mentor 2011;13(3):186–9.

8. Bell B, Thornton K. From promise to reality: achieving the value of an EHR: realizing the benefits of an EHR requires specific steps to establish goals, involve physicians and other key stakeholders, improve processes, and manage organizational change. Healthc financial Manag 2011; 65(2):51.

9. Suh KS, Sarojini S, Youssif M, et al. Tissue banking, bioinformatics, and electronic medical records: the front-end requirements for personalized medicine. J Oncol 2013;2013:368712–57.

10. Gauthier J, Vincent AT, Charette SJ, et al. A brief history of bioinformatics. Brief Bioinformatics 2019;20(6):1981–96.

11. Luscombe NM, Greenbaum D, Gerstein M. What is Bioinformatics? A Proposed Definition and Overview of the Field. Methods Inf Med 2001; 40(4):346–58.

12. Kulikowski CA, Shortliffe EH, Currie LM, et al. AMIA Board white paper: definition of biomedical informatics and specification of core competencies for graduate education in the discipline. J Am Med Inform Assoc : JAMIA. 2012;19(6): 931–8.

13. Friedman CP. A "fundamental theorem" of biomedical informatics. J Am Med Inform Assoc : JAMIA. 2009;16(2):169–70.

14. Gowd AK, Agarwalla A, Amin NH, et al. Construct validation of machine learning in the prediction of short-term postoperative complications following total shoulder arthroplasty. J Shoulder Elbow Surg 2019;28(12):e410–21.

15. Tajmir SH, Lee H, Shailam R, et al. Artificial intelligence-assisted interpretation of bone age radiographs improves accuracy and decreases variability. Skeletal Radiol 2018;48(2):275–83.

16. Cabitza F, Locoro A, Banfi G. Machine Learning in Orthopedics: A Literature Review. Front Bioeng Biotechnol 2018;6.

17. Kunze KN, Krivicich LM, Clapp IM, et al. Machine learning algorithms predict achievement of clinically significant outcomes after orthopaedic surgery: a systematic review. Arthroscopy 2022; 38(6):2090–105.

18. Lalehzarian SP, Gowd AK, Liu JN. Machine learning in orthopaedic surgery. World J Orthopedics 2021;12(9):685–99.

19. Myers TG, Ramkumar PN, Ricciardi BF, et al. Artificial Intelligence and Orthopaedics: An Introduction for Clinicians. J bone Jt Surg Am volume 2020;102(9):830–40.

20. Langton DJ, Bhalekar RM, Joyce TJ, et al. The influence of HLA genotype on the development of metal hypersensitivity following joint replacement. Commun Med 2022;2(1):73.

21. Mathew M T, Pai PS, Pourzal R, et al. Significance of tribocorrosion in biomedical applications: overview and current status. Adv Tribology 2009;2009: 1–12.

22. Carlson JCH, Citters DWV, Currier JH, et al. Femoral stem fracture and in vivo corrosion of retrieved modular femoral hips. J arthroplasty 2012;27(7):1389–96. e1381.

23. Collier JP, Surprenant VA, Jensen RE, et al. Corrosion between the components of modular femoral hip prostheses. J bone Jt Surg Br 1992;74(4): 511–7.

24. Cook SD, Barrack RL, Clemow AJT. Corrosion and wear at the modular interface of uncemented femoral stems. J bone Jt Surg Br volume 1994; 76(1):68–72.

25. Gilbert JL, Buckley CA, Jacobs JJ. In vivo corrosion of modular hip prosthesis components in mixed and similar metal combinations. The effect of crevice, stress, motion, and alloy coupling. J Biomed Mater Res 1993;27(12):1533–44.

26. Agins HJ, Alcock NW, Bansal M, et al. Metallic wear in failed titanium-alloy total hip replacements. A histological and quantitative analysis. J Bone And Joint Surg Am Volume 1988;70(3):347–56.

27. John Cooper H, Della Valle CJ, Berger RA, et al. Corrosion at the Head-Neck Taper as a Cause for Adverse Local Tissue Reactions After Total Hip Arthroplasty. J Bone And Joint Surg Am Volume 2012;94(18):1655–61.

28. Rodrigues DC, Urban RM, Jacobs JJ, et al. In vivo severe corrosion and hydrogen embrittlement of retrieved modular body titanium alloy hip-implants. J Biomed Mater Res B Appl Biomater 2009;88(1):206–19.

29. Gilbert JL. Corrosion in the Human Body: Metallic Implants in the Complex Body Environment. Corrosion 2017;73(12):1478–95.

30. Navarro M, Michiardi A, Castano O, et al. Biomaterials in orthopaedics. J R Soc Interf 2008;5(27): 1137–58.

31. Long M, Rack HJ. Titanium alloys in total joint replacement—a materials science perspective. Biomaterials 1998;19(18):1621–39.

32. Gilbert JL, Mali S, Urban RM, et al. In vivo oxide-induced stress corrosion cracking of Ti-6Al-4V in a neck–stem modular taper: Emergent behavior in a new mechanism of in vivo corrosion. J Biomed Mater Res B: Appl Biomater 2012; 100(2):584–94.

33. Goldberg JR, Gilbert JL, Jacobs JJ, et al. A multicenter retrieval study of the taper interfaces of modular hip prostheses. Clin Orthopaedics Relat Research® 2002;401:149–61.

34. Hamet P, Tremblay J. Artificial intelligence in medicine. Metab Clin Exp 2017;69:S36–40.

35. Coqueret G. In: Dixon Matthew F, Halperin Igor, Paul Bilokon, editors. Machine learning in finance: from theory to practiceVol 21. Routledge: Springer; 2021. p. 9–10. ISBN 978-3-030-41067-4. Paperback. In.

36. Wuest T, Weimer D, Irgens C, et al. Machine learning in manufacturing: advantages, challenges, and applications. Prod Manufacturing Res 2016;4(1):23–45.

37. Rajkomar A, Dean J, Kohane I. Machine Learning in Medicine. New Engl J Med 2019;380(14):1347–58.

38. Michalski RS, Carbonell JG, Mitchell TM. Machine learning: an artificial intelligence approach. Berlin/Heidelberg, Germany: Springer Science & Business Media; 2013.

39. Rosenblatt F. The perceptron: A probabilistic model for information storage and organization in the brain. Psychol Rev 1958;65(6):386–408.

40. LeCun Y, Touresky D, Hinton G, et al. A theoretical framework for back-propagation. Paper presented at: Proceedings of the 1988 connectionist models summer school, CMU, Pittsburgh, PA,1988.

41. LeCun Y, Bengio Y, Hinton G. Deep learning. Nature (London) 2015;521(7553):436–44.

42. Vouldimos A, Doulamis N, Doulamis A, et al. Deep learning for computer vision: a brief review. Comput intelligence Neurosci 2018;2018: 7068313–49.

43. Young T, Hazarika D, Poria S, et al. Recent trends in deep learning based natural language processing [Review Article]. IEEE Comput intelligence Mag 2018;13(3):55–75.

44. Jing Y, Bian Y, Hu Z, et al. Deep learning for drug design: an artificial intelligence paradigm for drug discovery in the big data Era. AAPS J 2018;20(3):58.

45. Min S, Lee B, Yoon S. Deep learning in bioinformatics. Brief Bioinformatics 2017;18(5):851–69.

46. Lai Z, Deng H. Medical Image Classification Based on Deep Features Extracted by Deep Model and

Statistic Feature Fusion with Multilayer Perceptron. Comput intelligence Neurosci 2018;2018: 2061513–6.

47. Olczak J, Fahlberg N, Maki A, et al. Artificial intelligence for analyzing orthopedic trauma radiographs: Deep learning algorithms-are they on par with humans for diagnosing fractures? Acta orthopaedica 2017;88(6):581–6.

48. Cortes C, Vapnik V. Support-vector networks. Machine Learn 1995;20(3):273–97.

49. Camlica Z, Tizhoosh HR, Khalvati F. Medical image classification via SVM using LBP features from saliency-based folded data. In: *2015 IEEE 14th international conference on machine learning and applications (ICMLA)*. IEEE; 2015. p. 128–32.

50. Agarwal S, Pandey GN. (2010, December). SVM based context awareness using body area sensor network for pervasive healthcare monitoring. In Proceedings of the First International Conference on Intelligent Interactive Technologies and Multimedia (pp. 271-278). December 27-30. Allahabad, India: Indian Institute of Information Technology; 2010.

51. Watanabe T, Kessler D, Scott C, et al. Disease prediction based on functional connectomes using a scalable and spatially-informed support vector machine. NeuroImage (Orlando, Fla) 2014;96: 183–202.

52. Smola AJ, Schölkopf B. A tutorial on support vector regression. Stat Comput 2004;14(3):199–222.

53. Ben-Hur A, Horn D, Siegelmann HT, et al. A support vector clustering method 2000.

54. Freund Y, Mason L. The alternating decision tree learning algorithm. Paper presented at: icml, 1999.

55. Jothi N, Rashid NAA, Husain W. Data Mining in Healthcare – A Review. Proced Comput Sci 2015; 72:306–13.

56. Azar AT, El-Metwally SM. Decision tree classifiers for automated medical diagnosis. Neural Comput Appl 2012;23(7–8):2387–403.

57. Rajendran P, Madheswaran M. Hybrid medical image classification using association Rule mining with decision tree algorithm. Ithaca: Cornell University Library, arXiv.org; 2010.

58. Fan C-Y, Chang P-C, Lin J-J, et al. A hybrid model combining case-based reasoning and fuzzy decision tree for medical data classification. Appl soft Comput 2011;11(1):632–44.

59. Tee JW, Rivers CS, Fallah N, et al. Decision tree analysis to better control treatment effects in spinal cord injury clinical research. J Neurosurg Spine 2019;31(4):464–72.

60. Boutsidis C, Drineas P, Mahoney MW. Unsupervised feature selection for the $ k $-means clustering problem. Adv Neural Inf Process Syst 2009;22.

61. Bottou L, Bengio Y. Convergence properties of the k-means algorithms. Adv Neural Inf Process Syst 1994;7.

62. Alsayat A, El-Sayed H. Efficient genetic K-Means clustering for health care knowledge discovery 2016.

63. Luong DTA, Chandola V. A k-means approach to clustering disease progressions. Paper presented 2017 IEEE Int Conf Healthc Inform (Ichi), 2017. August 23 2017 to August 26 2017, Park City, UT, USA

64. Ng H, Ong S, Foong K, et al. Medical image segmentation using k-means clustering and improved watershed algorithm. Paper presented at: 2006 IEEE southwest symposium on image analysis and interpretation, 2006. 26-28 March 2006, Denver, CO, USA.

65. Li J, Tang S, Zhang H, et al. Clustering of morphological fracture lines for identifying intertrochanteric fracture classification with Hausdorff distance–based K-means approach. Injury 2019;50(4):939–49.

66. Kop AM, Keogh C, Swarts E. Proximal Component Modularity in THA—At What Cost?: An Implant Retrieval Study. Clin orthopaedics Relat Res 2011;470(7):1885–94.

67. Fraitzl CR, Moya LE, Castellani L, et al. Corrosion at the Stem-Sleeve Interface of a Modular Titanium Alloy Femoral Component as a Reason for Impaired Disengagement. J arthroplasty 2011; 26(1):113–9. e111.

68. Rodrigues DC, Urban RM, Jacobs JJ, et al. In vivo severe corrosion and hydrogen embrittlement of retrieved modular body titanium alloy hip-implants. J Biomed Mater Res Part B: Appl Biomater 2009;88(1):206–19. The Japanese Society for Biomaterials, and The Australian Society for Biomaterials and the Korean Society for Biomaterials.

69. Urban RM, Gilbert JL, Jacobs JJ. Corrosion of Modular Titanium Alloy Stems in Cementless Hip Replacement. J ASTM Int 2005;2(10):1–10.

70. Gilbert JL, Jacobs JJ. The Mechanical and Electrochemical Processes Associated with Taper Fretting Crevice Corrosion: A Review. In: 100 barr harbor drive, PO box C70019428-2959. West Conshohocken, PA: ASTM International; 1997. p. 45–59.

71. Swaminathan V. Fretting crevice corrosion of metallic biomaterials: instrument development and materials analysis. Ann Arbor, MI: ProQuest Dissertations Publishing; 2012.

72. Viswanathan Swaminathan L, Gilbert J. Fretting corrosion of CoCrMo and Ti6Al4V interfaces. Biomaterials 2012;33(22):5487–503.

73. Mali S. Mechanically assisted crevice corrosion in metallic biomaterials: a review. Mater Technology 2016;31(12):732–9.

74. Jacobs JJ, Cooper HJ, Urban RM, et al. What Do We Know About Taper Corrosion in Total Hip Arthroplasty? J arthroplasty 2014;29(4):668–9.

75. Eltit F, Wang Q, Wang R. Mechanisms of Adverse Local Tissue Reactions to Hip Implants. Front Bioeng Biotechnol 2019;7:176.

76. Hall DJ, Pourzal R, Jacobs JJ. What Surgeons Need to Know About Adverse Local Tissue Reaction in Total Hip Arthroplasty. J arthroplasty 2020;35(6):S55–9.

77. Landolt D, Mischler S, Stemp M, et al. Third body effects and material fluxes in tribocorrosion systems involving a sliding contact. Wear 2004;256(5):517–24.

78. Barril S, Mischler S, Landolt D. Influence of fretting regimes on the tribocorrosion behaviour of Ti6Al4V in 0.9wt.% sodium chloride solution. Wear 2004;256(9–10):963–72.

79. Mischler S. Triboelectrochemical techniques and interpretation methods in tribocorrosion: A comparative evaluation. Tribology Int 2008;41(7):573–83.

80. Hall DJ, Pourzal R, Lundberg HJ, et al. Mechanical, chemical and biological damage modes within head-neck tapers of CoCrMo and Ti6Al4V contemporary hip replacements. J Biomed Mater Res Part B: Appl Biomater 2018;106(5):1672–85.

81. Kurtz MA, Khullar P, Gilbert JL. Cathodic activation and inflammatory species are critical to simulating in vivo Ti-6Al-4V selective dissolution. Acta Biomater 2022;149:399–409.

82. Prestat M, Vucko F, Holzer L, et al. Microstructural aspects of Ti6Al4V degradation in H2O2-containing phosphate buffered saline. Corrosion Sci 2021;190:109640.

83. Codirenzi AM. Large-scale Analysis and Automated Detection of Trunnion Corrosion on Hip Arthroplasty Devices. 2022.

84. Milimonfared R, Oskouei RH, Taylor M, et al. An intelligent system for image-based rating of corrosion severity at stem taper of retrieved hip replacement implants. Med Eng Phys 2018;61:13–24.

85. Milimonfared R. Development and implementation of an artificial intelligence system for assessing corrosion damage at stem taper of hip replacement implants: a retrieval study. Adelaide, South Australia: Flinders University, College of Science and Engineering; 2019.

86. Fessler RR. Pipeline corrosion. Report. Baker, Evanston, IL: US Department of Transportation Pipeline and Hazardous Materials Safety Administration; 2008.

87. Mansoori H, Mirzaee R, Esmaeilzadeh F, et al. Pitting corrosion failure analysis of a wet gas pipeline. Eng Fail Anal 2017;82:16–25.

88. Papavinasam S. Corrosion control in the oil and gas industry. Boston: Elsevier; 2014.

89. Alamri AH. Localized corrosion and mitigation approach of steel materials used in oil and gas pipelines – An overview. Eng Fail Anal 2020;116:104735.

90. Gilbert JL, Kubacki GW. Oxidative stress, inflammation, and the corrosion of metallic biomaterials: Corrosion causes biology and biology causes corrosion. In: Dziubla T, Butterfield DA, editors. Oxidative stress and biomaterials. Cambridge, MA: Elsevier; 2016. p. 59–88.

91. FDA U. Biological responses to metal implants. Silver spring (MD): Food and Drug Administration; 2019.

92. Jimenez-Come MJ, Turias IJ, Trujillo FJ. An automatic pitting corrosion detection approach for 316L stainless steel. Mater Des 2014;56:642–8.

93. Jimenez-Come MJ, Munoz E, Garcia R, et al. Pitting corrosion behaviour of austenitic stainless steel using artificial intelligence techniques. J Appl Logic 2012;10(4):291–7.

94. Jimenez-Come MJ, Munoz E, Garcia R, et al. Pitting Corrosion Detection of Austenitic Stainless Steel EN 1.4404 in MgCl2 solutions using a Machine Learning Approach. Paper presented 4th Manufacturing Eng Soc Int Conf (Mesic) 2012; 2011:21–3. Cadiz, SPAIN.

95. Wiegand MJ, Benton TZ, Gilbert JL. A fluorescent approach for detecting and measuring reduction reaction byproducts near cathodically-biased metallic surfaces: Reactive oxygen species production and quantification. Bioelectrochemistry 2019;129:235–41.

96. Morizet N, Godin N, Tang J, et al. Classification of acoustic emission signals using wavelets and Random Forests : Application to localized corrosion. Mech Syst Signal Process 2016;70-71:1026–37.

97. Rosen EM, Silverman DC. Corrosion prediction from polarization scans using an artificial neural network integrated with an expert system. Corrosion 1992;48(9):734–45.

98. Wiegand MJ, Shenoy AA, Littlejohn SE, et al. Sensing Localized Surface Corrosion Damage of CoCrMo Alloys and Modular Tapers of Total Hip Retrievals Using Nearfield Electrochemical Impedance Spectroscopy. ACS Biomater Sci Eng 2020;6(3):1344–54.

99. Shenoy A. Understanding Corrosion in Modular Acetabular Tapers: Retrieval Analysis, In Vitro Testing and Cell-Material Interactions, Clemson University Libraries.

100. Buck JA, Underhill PR, Morelli J, et al. Evaluation of machine learning tools for inspection of steam generator tube structures using pulsed eddy current. Paper presented AIP Conf Proc, 2017. Atlanta, Georgia, USA. 17–22 July 2016.

101. Gorji MB, de Pannemaecker A, Spevack S. Machine learning predicts fretting and fatigue key mechanical properties. Int J Mech Sci 2022;215.

102. Haviez L, Toscano R, Fourvy S, et al. Neural network for fretting wear modeling. Paper presented ICAART 2014 - Proc 6th Int Conf Agents Artif Intelligence, 2014. ESEO Angers, Loire Valley, France. 6-8 March 2014.

103. Kolodziejczyk T, Toscano R, Fouvry S, et al. Artificial intelligence as efficient technique for ball bearing fretting wear damage prediction. Wear 2010;268(1–2):309–15.

104. Kumar SA, Raman SGS, Narayanan TSNS, et al. Prediction of fretting wear behavior of surface mechanical attrition treated Ti-6Al-4V using artificial neural network. Mater Des 2013;49:992–9.

105. Nowell D, Nowell PW. A machine learning approach to the prediction of fretting fatigue life. Tribology Int 2020;141.

106. Ozarde AP, Narayan J, Yadav D, et al. Optimization of diesel engine's liner geometry to reduce head gasket's fretting damage. Sae Int J Engines 2021;14(1):81–97.

107. Qureshi W, Cura F, Mura A. Prediction of fretting wear in aero-engine spline couplings made of 42CrMo4. Proc Inst Mech Eng C, J Mech Eng Sci 2017;231(24):4684–92.

108. Sharma M, Bijwe J, Singh K. Studies for wear property correlation for carbon fabric-reinforced PES composites. Tribology Lett 2011;43(3):267–73.

109. Zhang G, Wang J, Chang S. Predicting running-in wear volume with a SVMR-based model under a small amount of training samples. Tribology Int 2018;128:349–55.

110. Bansal P, Zheng Z, Shao C, et al. Physics-informed machine learning assisted uncertainty quantification for the corrosion of dissimilar material joints. Reliability Eng Syst Saf 2022;227.

111. Kamrunnahar M, Urquidi-Macdonald M. Prediction of corrosion behaviour of Alloy 22 using neural network as a data mining tool. Corrosion Sci 2011;53(3):961–7.

112. Trasatti SP, Mazza F. Crevice corrosion: A neural network approach. Br Corrosion J 1996;31(2):105–12.

113. Agrawal R, Mukhopadhyay A. The use of machine learning and metaheuristic algorithm for wear performance optimization of AISI 1040 steel and investigation of corrosion resistance. Proc Inst Mech Eng J-Journal Eng Tribology 2022.

114. Ahuja SK, Shukla MK, Ravulakollu KK. Optimized deep learning framework for detecting pitting corrosion based on image segmentation. Int J Performability Eng 2021;17(7):627–37.

115. Ampazis N, Alexopoulos ND. Prediction of aircraft aluminum alloys tensile mechanical properties degradation using Support Vector Machines. Lecture Notes Computer Sci (including subseries Lecture Notes Artif Intelligence Lecture Notes Bioinformatics) 2010;6040:9–18.

116. Ben Seghier MEA, Keshtegar B, Taleb-Berrouane M, et al. Advanced intelligence frameworks for predicting maximum pitting corrosion depth in oil and gas pipelines. Process Saf Environ Prot 2021;147:818–33.

117. Boucherit MN, Arbaoui F. Pitting corrosion prediction from cathodic data: application of machine learning. Anti-Corrosion Methods Mater 2021;68(5):396–403.

118. Boucherit MN, Amzert SA, Arbaoui F, et al. Modelling input data interactions for the optimization of artificial neural networks used in the prediction of pitting corrosion. Anti-corrosion Methods Mater 2019;66(4):369–78.

119. Boukhari Y, Boucherit MN, Zaabat M, et al. Optimization of learning algorithms in the prediction of pitting corrosion. J Eng Sci Technology 2018;13(5):1153–64.

120. Boukhari Y, Boucherit MN, Zaabat M, et al. Artificial intelligence to predict inhibition performance of pitting corrosion. J Fundam Appl Sci 2017;9(1):308–22.

121. Chou J-S, Ngoc-Tri N, Chong WK. The use of artificial intelligence combiners for modeling steel pitting risk and corrosion rate. Eng Appl Artif Intelligence 2017;65:471–83.

122. Enikeev M, Enikeeva L, Maleeva M, et al. Machine learning in the problem of recognition of pitting corrosion on aluminum surfaces. Paper presented at: CEUR Workshop Proceedings. 2018. International Conference on "Information Technology and Nanotechnology" (ITNT-2018), Samara, Russia, April 24, 2018 - April 27, 2018

123. Hoang ND. Image processing-based pitting corrosion detection using metaheuristic optimized multi-level image thresholding and machine-learning approaches. Math Probl Eng 2020;2020.

124. Ji J, Zhang C, Kodikara J, et al. Prediction of stress concentration factor of corrosion pits on buried pipes by least squares support vector machine. Eng Fail Anal 2015;55:131–8.

125. Jesus Jimenez-Come M, de la Luz Martin M, Matres V. A support vector machine-based ensemble algorithm for pitting corrosion modeling of EN 1.4404 stainless steel in sodium chloride solutions. Mater Corrosion-Werkstoffe Und Korrosion 2019;70(1):19–27.

126. Kankar PK, Sharma SC, Harsha SP. Fault diagnosis of ball bearings using machine learning methods. Expert Syst Appl 2011;38(3):1876–86.

127. Kubisztal J, Kubisztal M, Haneczok G. Corrosion damage of 316L steel surface examined using statistical methods and artificial neural network. Mater Corrosion-Werkstoffe Und Korrosion 2020;71(11):1842–55.

128. Li Q, Wang J, Wang K, et al. Determination of Corrosion Types from Electrochemical Noise by

Gradient Boosting Decision Tree Method. Int J Electrochem Sci 2019;14(2):1516–28.

129. Li X, Kong X, Liu Z, et al. A Novel Framework for Early Pitting Fault Diagnosis of Rotating Machinery Based on Dilated CNN Combined With Spatial Dropout. Ieee Access 2021;9:29243–52.

130. Liu KC, Yang CH, Liu TI, et al. On-stream inspection for pitting corrosion defect of pressure vessels for intelligent and safe manufacturing. Int J Adv Manufacturing Technology 2017;91(5–8):1957–66.

131. Lu H, Peng H, Xu Z-D, et al. A Feature Selection-Based Intelligent Framework for Predicting Maximum Depth of Corroded Pipeline Defects. J Perform Constructed Facil 2022;36(5).

132. Pidaparti RM, Neblett EJ. Neural network mapping of corrosion induced chemical elements degradation in aircraft aluminum. Cmc-Computers Mater Continua 2007;5(1):1–9.

133. Pinto G, Amaral J, Pinheiro GRV, et al. Non-intrusive Internal Corrosion Characterization using the Potential Drop Technique for Electrical Mapping and Machine Learning. J Control Automation Electr Syst 2022;33(1):183–97.

134. Qu Z, Tang D, Wang Z, et al. Pitting Judgment Model Based on Machine Learning and Feature Optimization Methods. Front Mater 2021;8.

135. Roy N, Bhardwaj A, Kujur A, et al. Effect of heterogeneities on pitting potential of line pipe steels: An adaptive neuro-fuzzy approach. Corrosion Sci 2018;133:327–35.

136. Sanchez G, Aperador W, Ceron A. Corrosion grade classification: a machine learning approach. Indian Chem Engineer 2020;62(3):277–86.

137. Shin M-K, Jo WJ, Cha HM, et al. A study on the condition based maintenance evaluation system of smart plant device using convolutional neural network. J Mech Sci Technology 2020;34(6):2507–14.

138. Takara Y, Ozawa T, Yamaguchi M. Analysis of the elemental effects on the surface potential of aluminum alloy using machine learning. Jpn J Appl Phys 2022;61(SL).

139. Urda D, Marcos Luque R, Jesus Jimenez M, et al. A Constructive Neural Network to Predict Pitting Corrosion Status of Stainless Steel. Paper presented at: 12th International Work-Conference on Artificial Neural Networks. IWANN 2013;12–4. Puerto de la Cruz, SPAIN.

140. Wei X, Wen ZY, Xiao L, et al. Shear strength prediction of TCSWs with artificial pitting based on ANN. Paper presented at: Bridge Maintenance, Safety, Management, Life-Cycle Sustainability and Innovations - Proceedings of the 10th International Conference on Bridge Maintenance, Safety and Management. IABMAS 2020;2021.

141. Yajima A, Wang H, Liang RY, et al. A clustering based method to evaluate soil corrosivity for pipeline external integrity management. Int J Press Vessels Pip 2015;126:37–47.

142. Zhang Y, Zhou X, Shi H, et al. Corrosion pitting damage detection of rolling bearings using data mining techniques. IJMIC 2015;24(3):235–43.

Short-to Mid-Term Survivorship of a Patient-specific Unicompartmental Knee Arthroplasty Implant Cast from a Three-Dimensional Printed Mold

Alexandre Barbieri Mestriner, MD[a],
Brielle Antonelli, BA[b], Pierre-Emmanuel Schwab, MD[c],
Antonia F. Chen, MD, MBA[b], Todd Jones, BA[b],
Jakob Ackermann, MD[d], Gergo Bela Merkely, MD[b],
Jeffrey K. Lange, MD[b,*]

KEYWORDS

- Customized knee replacement • Unicompartmental knee replacement • New technology
- 3D printed implant

KEY POINTS

- Patient-specific unicompartmental knee arthroplasty (UKA) is a successful procedure with excellent survivorship at an average 4.5-year follow-up.
- Patient-specific UKA has comparable survivorship to conventional UKA at early- to mid-term follow-up.
- Further study is required to determine long-term outcomes of patient-specific UKA.

INTRODUCTION

Osteoarthritis (OA) affects over 30 million people[1] and is highly prevalent in the United States with current rates of OA more than twice what they were before the mid-twentieth century.[2] A subset of patients with OA of the knee experience OA that is confined predominantly to a single compartment, either medial, lateral, or patellofemoral. When surgery is indicated, unicompartmental knee replacement may be a good option for patients with predominantly unicompartmental involvement.[3]

The idea of unicompartmental knee arthroplasty (UKA) was first presented in the 1950s and with succeeding decades, this procedure has been modernized with advancements in technology and adapted surgical protocols to reach satisfactory patient outcomes.[3] UKA allows for the conservation of bone stock, spares the cruciate ligaments, and may be associated with reduced perioperative morbidity as compared with total knee arthroplasty (TKA) in some cases.[4] Benefits of UKA include the potential for accelerated recovery, superior functional outcomes, more natural knee kinematics, and lower postoperative complication rates as compared with total knee arthroplasty (TKA).[4–8] However, the rate of revision following UKA may be as great as three times higher compared

---

[a] Department of Orthopedics and Traumatology, Federal University of Sao Paulo - Paulista, School of Medicine, Sao Paulo, Brazil; [b] Department of Orthopedic Surgery, Brigham and Women's Hospital, Harvard Medical School, 75 Francis Street, Boston, MA, USA; [c] Tufts Medical Center, 800 Washington Street, Boston, MA, USA; [d] Department of Orthopedics, Balgrist University Hospital, University of Zurich, 8008 Zurich, Switzerland
* Corresponding author.
E-mail address: jlange1@bwh.harvard.edu

Orthop Clin N Am 54 (2023) 193–199
https://doi.org/10.1016/j.ocl.2022.12.001
0030-5898/23/© 2022 Elsevier Inc. All rights reserved.

with TKA.[9–12] Multiple factors can influence UKA survivorship, including patient, surgical, and implant factors.[13,14]

Implant design represents one area of focus for optimizing UKA survivorship.[11,15] One of the concerns surrounding conventional UKA implant design is the potential for anatomic mismatch leading to early failure, either by persistent pain due to oversizing and impingement or by early loosening and subsidence due to undersizing.[16–18] Individualized UKA addresses sizing concerns by promoting a more accurate anatomic fit to individual joint geometry. Previous research has shown that patient-specific implants provide improved cortical rim surface area coverage, less overhang and undercoverage,[11] and greater overall tibial bone coverage as compared with conventional implants.[19] In addition, patient-specific implants preserve femoral bone and create more equal bone-implant stress distribution on the bone-implant interface that may reduce chances of early implant loosening.[20,21]

In 2012, the second generation of a UKA implant cast from a three-dimensional (3D) printed mold was introduced into the market (iUni, ConforMIS, Inc. Billerica, Massachusetts). Although long-term follow-up is necessary to assess the durability of any implant, short-term follow-up is imperative to monitor implant performance before long-term results are available. The purpose of this study was to determine survivorship and complication rates associated with implantation of a single design UKA implant cast from a 3D printed mold at short-to mid-term follow-up.

MATERIALS AND METHODS
Patient Selection
We performed a retrospective review of all patients that underwent UKA with an implant cast from a 3D printed mold (iUNI; ConforMIS, Inc; Burlington, Massachusetts) between September 2012 and October 2015 by a single surgeon at a single institution with approval from the Institutional Review Board (IRB). Data collected included patients' age at the time of procedure, sex, laterality (left, right or bilateral), knee compartment (medial or lateral), primary diagnosis, comorbidities, smoking status, body mass index (BMI), and concomitant procedures. Patients with incomplete data or who underwent a concomitant procedure were excluded.

Surgical Technique
All UKAs were performed by a single high-volume joint replacement surgeon. Medial UKAs were performed through a short medial parapatellar approach, whereas lateral UKAs were performed through a short lateral parapatellar approach. Postoperative alignment goal was restoration of individual alignment before osteoarthritic changes based on soft tissue tension in extension with more laxity (2 to 3 mm) lateral compared with medial (1 to 2 mm) facilitated by patient-specific cutting guides.

Complications and Osteoarthritis Progression
All postoperative complications were recorded. Progression of OA in unresurfaced compartments was also reported. Rate of conversion to TKA and rate of reoperation for any reason were reported separately.

Knee Range of Motion
During each appointment, knee ROM was routinely measured. Pre- and postoperative measurements were collected to determine final ROM improvement.

Imaging Analysis
Anteroposterior full-length weightbearing radiographs were used to evaluate lower limb alignment. Alignment was measured on preoperative and postoperative images using the hip-knee-ankle (HKA) angle. The HKA angle was defined as the angle between the following two lines: a line drawn from the center of the femoral head to the center of the knee, and a line drawn from the center of the knee to the midpoint on the talar dome. A negative HKA angle indicated varus alignment and a positive HKA angle indicated valgus alignment.[22] We considered values between -3° to 3° to be neutral.[22] All measurements were performed using the PACS system (Centricity, General Electric Healthcare, Boston, Massachusetts).

Statistical Data Analysis
Kaplan–Meyer survival curve was used in survivorship calculation for both medial and lateral UKA implants using conversion to TKA and reoperation for any reason as two separate endpoints. Paired T-test was used for evaluating and comparing pre- and postoperative knee ROM and alignment. Chi-square test was used to assess the relationship between the involved compartment (medial or lateral) and complication or disease progression rates. Statistical analysis was performed with SPSS for Mac (version 22.0, SPSS, Chicago, Illinois). Significance was set at $P < .05$.

RESULTS

Our final study cohort included 105 knees (92 patients) with a mean follow-up of 4.5 ± 2.2 years (range 0.4 to 7.7 years). Ninety-four knees (89.5%) had a minimum 2-year follow-up. Mean age at the time of surgery was 61.8 ± 9.1 years. Most of the UKAs were indicated for unicompartmental knee OA (98%). Eighty-eight knees (83.8%) underwent medial UKA and 17 knees (16.2%) underwent lateral UKA. Demographic data of the final analytical cohort are presented in Table 1.

Medial and lateral compartment UKA survivorship free from conversion to TKA were 98.8% and 94.1%, respectively, at final follow-up (Table 2). Reoperation rate for any reason was 2.9% (three knees), resulting in an overall survivorship free from reoperation of 97.1% in our cohort of 105 knees (see Table 2). One medial implant failed within the first 2 years after surgery due to tibial component loosening as a result of a mechanical fall directly onto the knee at 4 months postoperatively and was converted to a TKA. One lateral implant failed 6 years after surgery due to pain, buckling, and effusion which required conversion to TKA where bone loss of the lateral femoral condyle was found intraoperatively. The third reoperation was due to a substantial hemarthrosis after a medial UKA that required drainage. One patient had persistent debilitating pain at 14 months after the surgery but had not undergone reoperation at the final follow-up. During the follow-up period, three patients died due to reasons unrelated to the procedure or implant.

In cases of preoperative varus alignment ($n = 88$; preoperative mean HKA angle $-8.3° ± 3.6°$), the mean alignment correction was $8.5° ± 4.1°$ ($P = .003$). Patients with preoperative valgus alignment ($n = 17$; preoperative mean HKA $4.0° ± 2.4°$) underwent a mean alignment correction of $-1.4° ± 1.8°$ ($P = .031$). Postoperative ROM was significantly improved by $8.4° ± 12.0°$ ($P = .004$) (Table 3).

Overall complication rates are recorded in Table 4. Nine patients (8.6%) experienced perioperative complications including five wound healing complications treated nonsurgically (local wound care with or without antibiotics), one hemarthrosis treated nonsurgically, one report of neuropathic pain over the surgical scar, one report of functionally limiting pain, and one report of loosening due to trauma at 14 months after surgery treated nonsurgically. Seventeen knees (16.2%) presented with radiographic evidence of OA progression of unresurfaced compartments at final follow-up. Of these, four patients (24%) reported occasional symptoms such as pain and effusion that did not limit function. No patients with OA progression required revision procedures during the follow-up period. We found no significant association between laterality of the involved compartment and complication rates or OA progression rates ($P = .57$; $P = .66$, respectively).

Table 1 Demographics of patients who underwent unicondylar knee arthroplasty with a patient-specific implant cast from a 3D printed mold	
Age at time of surgery (years)	61.8 (±9.1)
Sex	
Male	44 (47.8)
Female	48 (52.2)
Laterality	
Right	60 (57.1)
Left	45 (42.9)
Diagnosis	
Osteoarthritis	103 (98.0)
Osteonecrosis	1 (1.0)
Rheumatoid arthritis	1 (1.0)
Smoking status	
Smoker	8 (8.7)
Former smoker	38 (41.3)
Non-smoker	46 (50.0)
Deformity	
Varus	88 (83.8)
Valgus	17 (16.2)
UKA compartment	
Medial	88 (83.8)
Lateral	17 (16.2)
BMI (kg/m^2)	30.2 (±6.1)

Abbreviation: BMI, body mass index.
Continuous variables are reported as mean (standard deviation). Categorical variables are reported as *N* (percentage of total cohort).

DISCUSSION

In our cohort of 105 knees, we showed excellent survivorship of both medial and lateral patient-specific UKA implant cast from a 3D printed mold at mean 4.5-year follow-up, with a reoperation rate for any reason of 2.9%. Postoperative limb alignment correction and ROM improvement were statistically significant. The rate of radiographic OA progression was 16% at final follow-up; however, only 24% of those patients

Table 2
Reoperation rates are reported overall and specifically for conversion to total knee arthroplasty in patients who underwent unicompartmental knee arthroplasty with a patient-specific implant cast from a 3D printed mold

Replaced Compartment of the Knee	Total Number of Knees	Number of Reoperations for Any Reason	Survivorship Free From Reoperation		Number of Knees Revised to TKA	Survivorship Free From Conversion to TKA	
			N	%		N	%
Medial	88	2	86	97.7	1	87	98.8
Lateral	17	1	16	94.1	1	16	94.1
Overall	105	3	102	97.1	2	103	98.1

Abbreviation: TKA, total knee arthroplasty.

complained of symptoms and those symptoms were not functionally limiting. Since much of the published literature regarding OA progression following UKA focuses on revision rates, our reported OA progression rate is not exactly comparable. However, at least the percentage of patients with symptomatic OA progression in our cohort (4%) is within range of the published revision rates for OA progression following UKA of 2% to 8%.[23]

Our results compare favorably with the results of previously reported short-term survivorship of conventional unicompartmental knee replacement implants. For instance, Goodfellow and colleagues[24] reported the results of 103 conventional UKAs (76 medial and 27 lateral) performed by a single surgeon with an average follow-up of 3 years, demonstrating a cumulative survivorship rate of 91% and 93% for medial and lateral implants, respectively. Middleton and colleagues[25] reported the results of 129 conventional UKAs at a mean 5.5-year follow-up, demonstrating a survivorship of 90%. In a large cohort of 909 robotically-assisted UKAs, the overall survivorship was found to be 96% at a mean follow-up of 2.5 years.[26] Both our overall survivorship rate free from conversion to TKA of 98.1% and

overall survivorship rate free from any reoperation of 97.1% are favorable compared with these other cohorts; however, the average follow-up of 4.5 years is relatively short (range 0.4 to 7.7 years).

There are few studies reporting outcomes following patient-specific unicompartmental knee implants for UKA. Demange and colleagues[19] evaluated 33 patient-specific lateral UKAs and showed improved tibial coverage when compared with standard lateral UKAs. The authors reported a survivorship of 97% at an average follow-up of 3.1 years and excellent short-term clinical results with clinically meaningful improvements in the Knee Society score after surgery. Separately, using a computer-aided design model and virtually performed surgeries, Carpenter and colleagues[15] compared five off-the-shelf medial and lateral UKA implants to patient-specific UKA and showed superior cortical bone coverage and a better fit on the tibial plateau of the custom-made implant (77% vs 43% medially and 60% vs 37% laterally), resulting in reduced overhang and undercoverage. Koeck and colleagues,[27] in a prospective study, evaluated the lower limb axis correction in 32 knees following patient-specific medial

Table 3
Preoperative and postoperative coronal alignment and range of motion are reported for patients who underwent unicompartmental knee arthroplasty with a patient-specific implant cast from a 3D printed mold

	Preoperative	Postoperative	Correction	*P-value*
Varus deformity, °	−8.3 (±3.6)	0.2 (±3.6)	8.5 (±4.1)	.003
Valgus deformity, °	4.0 (±2.4)	2.6 (±1.1)	− 1.4 (±1.8)	.031
Range of motion, °	124.1 (±12.7)	132.5 (±4.9)	8.4 (±12.0)	.004

Variables are reported as mean (standard deviation). *P*-values represent comparisons between preoperative and postoperative variables; $P < .05$ is considered statistically significant. Negative values indicate varus alignment. Positive values indicate valgus alignment.

Table 4
Complications, osteoarthritis progression, and reoperation rates for patients who underwent unicompartmental knee arthroplasty with a patient-specific implant cast from a 3D printed mold with minimum 2 y follow-up

		N (%)	Medial UKA	Lateral UKA
Complications				
	Wound-healing complications	5 (4.8)	4	1
	Hemarthrosis	1 (1.0)	–	1
	Neuropatic pain over scar	1 (1.0)	1	–
	Loosening as a result of trauma	1 (1.0)	1	–
	Functionally limiting pain	1 (1.0)	1	–
OA progression		17 (16.2)	14	3
	Symptomatic (pain and effusion)	4 (3.8)	3	1
	Non-symptomatic	13 (12.4)	11	2
Reoperations		3 (2.9)	2	1
	Conversion to TKA	2 (1.9)	1	1
	Hemarthrosis requiring evacuation	1 (1.0)	1	–

Abbreviations: OA, osteoarthritis; TKA, total knee arthroplasty; UKA, unicompartmental knee arthroplasty.
Complications, OA progression, and reoperations are reported. The column entitled N (%) represents the number of complications reported and percentage of the whole cohort.

UKA. The authors showed precise postoperative lower limb axis correction in the coronal plane overall, precise establishment of the medial proximal tibial angle, and precise maintenance of the tibial slope. In addition, the authors showed precise postoperative implant positioning in both anteroposterior and mediolateral projections. Compared with other studies investigating the outcomes of patient-specific UKA implants cast from a 3D printed mold, our cohort represents a larger number UKAs and shows comparable short-term survivorship and limb alignment correction.

This study has several limitations. First, the lack of a control group allows only for a comparison with other implants through the available literature. Second, although we collected patient-reported outcomes, our response rate was too low to report meaningful results (less than 30%), and we therefore did not include these in our analysis. Third, we report only short-term results, and longer follow-up is imperative to evaluate the durability of this implant. In addition, although it may be viewed as a limitation that we included all cases during the selected study period, even before the typical 2-year minimum follow-up milestone, we believe the inclusion of all cases is important to present the most accurate snapshot of available outcome data regarding this novel implant, which has no significant follow-up to date in the literature.

SUMMARY

Unicompartmental knee arthroplasty using a patient-specific UKA implant cast from a 3D printed mold resulted in excellent survivorship of 97.1% overall at an average 4.5-year follow-up. To the best of our knowledge, this is the first report of short-term survivorship of this implant and represents the largest cohort of 3D-printed patient-specific UKAs In clinical reports. Longer-term studies are required to further investigate the performance and durability of this implant.

CLINICS CARE POINTS

- Patient-specific unicompartmental knee arthroplasty (UKA) is a successful procedure with excellent survivorship at an average 4.5-year follow-up.

- Patient-specific UKA has comparable survivorship to conventional UKA at early- to mid-term follow-up.

- Further study is required to determine long-term outcomes of patient-specific UKA.

DISCLOSURE

Conformis (Consultant - Education), OnPoint Knee (Scientific Advisory Board), Aesculap

(Consultant), SLACK Incorporated (Royalties), American Association of Hip and Knee Surgeons (Committee Member), UpToDate (Royalties), Stryker (Royalties), Adaptive Phage Therapeutics (Consultant), Avanos (Consultant), BICMD (Consultant), Convatec (Consultant), Ethicon (Consultant), GLG (Consultant), Guidepoint (Consultant), Heraeus (Consultant), IrriMax (Consultant), Pfizer (Consultant), Hyalex (Stock), Irrimax (Stock), Joint Purification Systems (Stock), Sonoran (Stock), and IlluminOss (Stock)

REFERENCES

1. Cisternas MG, Murphy L, Sacks JJ, et al. Alternative methods for defining osteoarthritis and the impact on estimating prevalence in a us population-based survey. Arthritis Care Res (Hoboken) 2016;68(5): 574–80.
2. Wallace IJ, Worthington S, Felson DT, et al. Knee osteoarthritis has doubled in prevalence since the mid-20th century. Proc Natl Acad Sci U S A 2017; 114(35):9332–6.
3. Bruni D, Iacono F, Akkawi I, et al. Unicompartmental knee replacement: a historical overview. Joints 2013;1(2):45–7.
4. Mohammad HR, Strickland L, Hamilton TW, et al. Long-term outcomes of over 8,000 medial oxford phase 3 unicompartmental knees-a systematic review. Acta Orthop 2018;89(1):101–7.
5. Lyons MC, MacDonald SJ, Somerville LE, et al. Unicompartmental versus total knee arthroplasty database analysis: is there a winner? Clin Orthop Relat Res 2012;470(1):84–90.
6. Dalury DF, Fisher DA, Adams MJ, et al. Unicompartmental knee arthroplasty compares favorably to total knee arthroplasty in the same patient. Orthopedics 2009;32(4).
7. Hopper GP, Leach WJ. Participation in sporting activities following knee replacement: total versus unicompartmental. Knee Surg Sports Traumatol Arthrosc 2008;16(10):973–9.
8. Kim KT, Lee S, Lee JI, et al. Analysis and Treatment of Complications after Unicompartmental Knee Arthroplasty. Knee Surg Relat Res 2016;28(1):46–54.
9. Liddle AD, Judge A, Pandit H, et al. Adverse outcomes after total and unicompartmental knee replacement in 101,330 matched patients: a study of data from the National Joint Registry for England and Wales. Lancet 2014;384(9952):1437–45.
10. Chawla H, van der List JP, Christ AB, et al. Annual revision rates of partial versus total knee arthroplasty: A comparative meta-analysis. Knee 2017; 24(2):179–90.
11. W-Dahl A, Robertsson O, Lidgren L, et al. Unicompartmental knee arthroplasty in patients aged less than 65. Acta Orthop 2010;81(1):90–4.
12. Robertsson O, Bizjajeva S, Fenstad AM, et al. Knee arthroplasty in Denmark, Norway and Sweden. A pilot study from the Nordic Arthroplasty Register Association. Acta Orthop 2010;81(1):82–9.
13. Lau RL, Perruccio AV, Gandhi R, et al. The role of surgeon volume on patient outcome in total knee arthroplasty: a systematic review of the literature. BMC Musculoskelet Disord 2012;13:250.
14. Liddle AD, Pandit H, Judge A, et al. Optimal usage of unicompartmental knee arthroplasty: a study of 41,986 cases from the National Joint Registry for England and Wales. Bone Joint J 2015;97-B(11): 1506–11.
15. Carpenter DP, Holmberg RR, Quartulli MJ, et al. Tibial plateau coverage in UKA: a comparison of patient specific and off-the-shelf implants. J Arthroplasty 2014;29(9):1694–8.
16. Schotanus MG, Sollie R, van Haaren EH, et al. A radiological analysis of the difference between MRI- and CT-based patient-specific matched guides for total knee arthroplasty from the same manufacturer: a randomised controlled trial. Bone Joint J 2016;98-B(6):786–92.
17. Gudena R, Pilambaraei MA, Werle J, et al. A safe overhang limit for unicompartmental knee arthroplasties based on medial collateral ligament strains: an in vitro study. J Arthroplasty 2013;28(2): 227–33.
18. Chau R, Gulati A, Pandit H, et al. Tibial component overhang following unicompartmental knee replacement–does it matter? Knee 2009;16(5): 310–3.
19. Demange MK, von Keudell A, Probst C, et al. Patient-specific implants for lateral unicompartmental knee arthroplasty. Int Orthop 2015;39(8):1519–26.
20. Fitzpatrick C, Fitzpatrick D, Lee J, et al. Statistical design of unicompartmental tibial implants and comparison with current devices. Knee 2007;14(2): 138–44.
21. Harrysson OL, Hosni YA, Nayfeh JF. Custom-designed orthopedic implants evaluated using finite element analysis of patient-specific computed tomography data: femoral-component case study. BMC Musculoskelet Disord 2007;8:91.
22. Abu-Rajab RB, Deakin AH, Kandasami M, et al. Hip-knee-ankle radiographs are more appropriate for assessment of post-operative mechanical alignment of total knee arthroplasties than standard ap knee radiographs. J Arthroplasty 2015;30(4): 695–700.
23. Jennings JM, Kleeman-Forsthuber LT, Bolognesi MP. Medial unicompartmental arthroplasty of the knee. J Am Acad Orthop Surg 2019; 27:166–76.
24. Goodfellow JW, Kershaw CJ, Benson MK, et al. The Oxford Knee for unicompartmental osteoarthritis.

The first 103 cases. J Bone Joint Surg Br 1988;70(5): 692–701.

25. Middleton SWF, Schranz PJ, Mandalia VI, et al. The largest survivorship and clinical outcomes study of the fixed bearing Stryker Triathlon Partial Knee Replacement - A multi-surgeon, single centre cohort study with a minimum of two years of follow-up. Knee 2018;25(4):732–6.

26. Pearle AD, van der List JP, Lee L, et al. Survivorship and patient satisfaction of robotic-assisted medial unicompartmental knee arthroplasty at a minimum two-year follow-up. Knee 2017;24(2):419–28.

27. Koeck FX, Beckmann J, Luring C, et al. Evaluation of implant position and knee alignment after patient-specific unicompartmental knee arthroplasty. Knee 2011;18(5):294–9.

Pediatrics

Intraoperative Navigation and Robotics in Pediatric Spinal Deformity

Zachary R. Diltz, MD[a,b,c], Benjamin J. Sheffer, MD[a,b,c],*

KEYWORDS

- 3D navigation • Robotics • Machine vision • Spinal deformity • Pediatrics

KEY POINTS

- Intraoperative navigation uses an intraoperative computed tomography (CT) scan or a series of fluoroscopic images to provide a 3D reconstruction of patient anatomy with real-time tracking of surgical instruments.
- Robotic arms place drill sleeves at templated trajectories for pedicle screw placement intraoperatively.
- Advantages of navigation and robotics include potential for increased pedicle screw accuracy particularly in patients having complex anatomy with deformity, decreased surgeon radiation exposure, and minimally invasive applications.
- Potential limitations include cost, perceived difficulties with operating workflow, and inaccurate registrations.
- Machine vision guidance is a relatively newer technology that uses no radiation and is able to quickly perform registration with recent evidence demonstrating similar accuracy of pedicle screw placement and improved operating room (OR) workflow compared with CT-based navigation and traditional fluoroscopy.

INTRODUCTION

Knowledge of appropriate anatomy is critical for surgeons but the development of intraoperative 3-dimensional (3D) imaging and navigation systems has supplemented this to improve spatial orientation during surgery. Various systems have been developed that allow for real-time 3D imaging and surgical instrument tracking during surgery for use in multiple areas within orthopedics including trauma, arthroplasty, arthroscopy, tumor, and spine.[1] Both navigation and robotics rely on radiographic imaging and/or topographic information to generate the production of a stereotactic field that is then used by the surgeon with the hopes of improving accuracy and reproducibility of a surgical procedure to minimize risk to the patient.[2]

The use of stereotaxy in surgery was first described by Horsley and Clarke in 1908, in which they attached a frame to the skull of a monkey to target intracranial lesions.[3] The use of computed tomography (CT) merged with advances in complex computer processing modernized this concept. By the late 1990s, the use of image guidance was described in spine surgery for placement of lumbar pedicle screws[4] and in computer-assisted total knee arthroplasty.[5] The range and number of available technologies for imaging, navigation, and robotics for applications in spinal surgery continues to increase.[6] This review will summarize

[a] Department of Orthopedic Surgery, LeBonheur Children's Hospital, 848 Adams Avenue, Memphis, TN 38103, USA; [b] Department of Orthopedic Surgery, Campbell Clinic, University of Tennessee Health Science Center, 1211 Union Avenue, Memphis, TN 38104, USA; [c] Campbell Clinic Orthopedics, 1400 South Germantown Road, Germantown, TN 38138, USA
* Corresponding author. Campbell Clinic Orthopedics, 1400 South Germantown Road, Germantown, TN 38138.
E-mail address: bsheffer@campbellclinic.com

Orthop Clin N Am 54 (2023) 201–207
https://doi.org/10.1016/j.ocl.2022.11.005
0030-5898/23/© 2022 Elsevier Inc. All rights reserved.

the perceived benefits as well as potential limitations of these new technologies because they relate specifically to pediatric deformity, as well as report the most recent literature available for the newer machine vision navigation technology.

Image Guidance Navigation and Robotics

Navigation can be used in passive or active systems. In passive navigation systems, the surgeon maintains complete control of all aspects of the surgical operation. There are no restraints placed or manual guidance given during surgery. However, there is real-time navigated tracking of surgical instruments including awls, pedicle finders, taps, and screwdrivers (**Fig. 1**). The theoretical advantage lies in the surgeon being able to use this information to more easily and accurately place pedicle screws and other hardware, such as cages. In contrast, active navigation or robotic systems involve the performance of a portion of the procedure by an automated robotic arm. For example, a surgeon plans pedicle screw trajectories based on preoperative imaging and an automated robotic arm guides a drill sleeve to this trajectory intraoperatively. Thus, a major difference between the two is the additional step of preplanning screw trajectories when using active systems. An example of the intraoperative OR setup for a navigation system is demonstrated in **Fig. 2**.

There are several options available for intraoperative image acquisition. Current second-generation 3D fluoroscopic scanning options have improved image quality and wider field of views as compared with first-generation scanners. A reference array is placed on the patient intraoperatively before image acquisition to allow for integration with navigation platforms. These arrays are typically clamped onto a spinous process or placed into the posterior superior iliac spine or other static landmark at surgeon discretion. Navigation allows for real-time tracking of surgical instruments by using infrared light produced by battery-powered instruments or reflective spheres. Another navigation system that does not integrate with an intraoperative fluoroscopic imaging system but instead uses machine vision cameras is 7D Surgical (**Fig. 3**). The machine vision cameras in this system coregister bony anatomy after surgical dissection is completed intraoperatively with a preoperative CT scan in order to produce a 3D reconstruction of patient anatomy. Thus, there is no radiation used during intraoperative registration, instead using visible light that is similar to facial recognition technology in mobile phones.

Current-generation robotic systems assist with screw placement through an active robotic arm that is mounted to a mobile base or the OR table itself. These systems can be integrated to either preoperative CT, intraoperative CT, or 2D fluoroscopy and are compatible with integrated navigation. This has the advantage of being able to judge screw depth and navigate prostheses and implants.

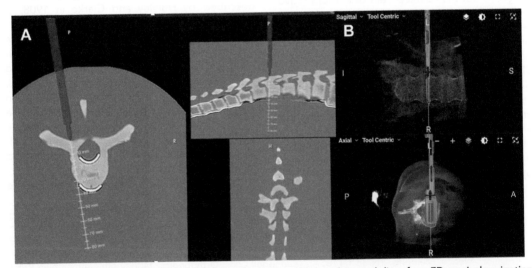

Fig. 1. Navigated tracking of surgical instruments. (*A*) Axial, sagittal, and coronal slices from 7D surgical navigation demonstrating real-time feedback of instruments in relation to the bony reconstruction of patient's anatomy. (*B*) Sagittal (*top*) and axial (*bottom*) reconstructions demonstrating tracking of a lateral interbody cage as it is placed into the intervertebral disc space. L, tracking from 7D surgical; R, sagittal and axial cuts from globus excelsius demonstrating tracking of lateral interbody cage.

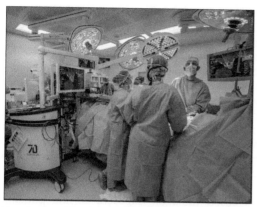

Fig. 2. Example of the intraoperative OR navigation setup. The mobile base of the system is positioned at the foot of the bed with the machine vision camera positioned overhead with a clear line of sight to the patient's anatomy and the surgical instruments for navigation.

Advantages of Navigation and Robotics in Spinal Surgery

There are several theoretical advantages to the use of image guidance in spinal surgery. Three main areas of interest include increased pedicle

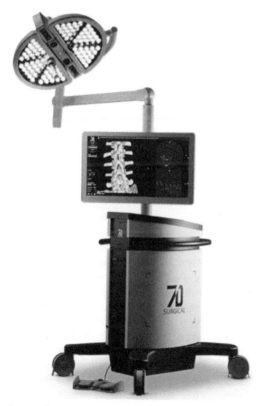

Fig. 3. The 7D Surgical with machine vision camera. Rather than fluoroscopic imaging, this system uses visible light for reconstruction of bony anatomy.

screw accuracy when compared with traditional freehand technique, decreased radiation exposure to the surgical team, and potential for increased application of minimally invasive techniques.

Pedicle screw accuracy: Pedicle screw fixation is a common technique in thoracolumbar fusions for spinal deformity, trauma, and other pathologic conditions. Techniques for freehand placement as well as using 2D fluoroscopy are well described.[7,8] However, there is concern over placement accuracy, especially in the thoracic spine with narrower pedicles creating a lower margin for error.[9] Moreover, placement can be more difficult in severe deformity and scoliosis due to altered anatomy. Breach rates using freehand techniques and 2D fluoroscopy have been reported between 1.5% and 21%.[8,10–13]

Image guidance and robotics purportedly have the benefit of increased accuracy of pedicle screws given the ability to use 3D reconstructions and navigated feedback of instruments during placement. There is a strong body of evidence supporting the use of image-guided navigation for this purpose. A randomized controlled trial by Laine and colleagues[14] examined pedicle screw placement by conventional techniques versus with the assistance of computer-assisted image guidance. There was a significantly lower pedicle perforation rate in the image guidance group (4.6%) versus the conventional technique (13.4%). Another international, multicenter prospective registry reported accuracy of their pedicle screw placement using intraoperative CT-based navigation at 97.5%.[15] About 1.8% of breaches was identified and corrected intraoperatively.

Robotic pedicle screw placement has shown mixed results in the literature. In a retrospective review, Molliqaj and colleagues[16] found a higher rate of accurate screw placement in the robot-assisted group (93.4%) when compared with the freehand fluoroscopic group (88.9%). In a randomized controlled trial performed by Ringel and colleagues[17] comparing robot-assisted placement to traditional technique, they found a higher rate of malposition in the robot group (15%) compared with the traditional freehand technique group (7%). In this study, 7% of robot-assisted screws had to be converted to freehand technique, highlighting the need for proficiency and knowledge of traditional techniques as a backup in cases of malfunction.

Navigation and robotics can also be a valuable tool for pedicle screw placement in the setting of complex anatomy in patients with deformity. Baldwin and colleagues[18] performed a systematic review of CT-based navigation in pediatric scoliosis surgery. They found screws placed with navigation were 3 times more likely to acceptable, 2 times as likely to be perfect, and only one-third as likely to be potentially unsafe when compared with screws placed with 2D fluoroscopy. Similarly, Baky and colleagues[19] found a lower rate of malpositioned pedicle screws when using CT navigation (1.0%) versus the fluoroscopic group (3.3%). There was a 3.6% rate of return to the OR for malposition in the fluoroscopic group while no patient required return to the OR in the CT navigation group. Gonzalez and colleagues[20] reported on their first 40 cases using robotic-assisted technology for the treatment of pediatric spinal deformity. Of 314 screws placed, they had a 98.7% accuracy rate and no clinically relevant screw complications. The effectiveness of CT-guided navigation has also been investigated specifically in prepubertal pediatric patients. This is of particular interest because young patients have smaller pedicle size and frequently complex deformity, which can lead to increased rates of screw malposition.[21] Luo and colleagues[22] investigated patients aged younger than 10 years undergoing pedicle screw placement using CT-guided navigation and found a 97.8% accuracy rate. Additionally, there is potential for an increased pedicle screw density in spinal deformity patients because CT-based navigation can allow for the placement of screws where laminar hooks or wires would have to be placed when using traditional techniques.[23] This is important because screws are stronger than hooks or wires.

Recently, multiple studies have investigated outcomes of pedicle screw placement using 7D Surgical's machine vision system. These have shown noninferiority in pedicle screw accuracy when compared with traditional techniques as well as CT-based navigation. Dorilio and colleagues[24] found no significant difference in pedicle screw accuracy using machine vision image guidance when compared with traditional 2D fluoroscopy (94.2% vs 96.6%). Malham and colleagues[25] performed a randomized controlled trial comparing pedicle screw placement using machine vision image guidance to traditional CT-based navigation. Pedicle screw accuracy was greater in the machine vision group (98.1% vs 97.3%) but there were no breaches greater than 2 mm in either group.

Decreased Radiation Exposure: Another benefit of image guidance and navigation lies in potential for decreased radiation exposure to the surgical team intraoperatively compared with traditional 2D fluoroscopy. With the use of CT-based navigation, the surgeon can leave the room while the scan of the operative field takes place, which decreases radiation exposure because the spine is instrumented using real-time feedback from the 3D reconstruction without the need for fluoroscopic imaging. Mendelsohn and colleagues[26] found a 2.5-fold decrease in surgeon radiation exposure during surgeries performed using CT-based navigation when compared with traditional fluoroscopic controls.

However, this often comes at the cost of increased radiation exposure to the patient. The standard radiation dose for the CT-scan used in CT-based protocols is 5.6 mSv, or the equivalent of 280 chest radiographs.[27] However, protocols have been developed to decrease the radiation dose to as low as 0.8 mSv.[28] Exposure when using fluoroscopy varies greatly depending on patient anatomy and surgeon experience but has been shown to be less than the cumulative preoperative and intraoperative dose when using CT-based navigation.[26,29,30]

An advantage of machine vision technology for navigation is decreased radiation exposure to the surgical team. When using machine vision, intraoperative fluoroscopy using ionizing radiation is needed to check levels and confirm pedicle screws at the end of the case. However, intraoperative image acquisition for navigation is performed with projected visible light rather than ionizing radiation. The literature has shown decreased radiation exposure using this technology. Dorilio and colleagues[24] found that patients undergoing spine surgery using 3D machine vision had reduced radiation exposure when compared with surgery using traditional 2D fluoroscopy, although this did not reach statistical significance. Similarly, Malham and colleagues[25] investigated radiation exposure in machine vision cases compared with traditional CT-based 3D navigation. They found a significant reduction of 94.3% in intraoperative fluoroscopy time and 97.8% in radiation dose in the machine vision group. Further studies will be needed to look at overall radiation exposure to the patient as machine vision systems still require a preoperative CT scan to be performed, which is coupled to the exposed intraoperative vertebral bodies captured by the stereoscopic cameras.

Minimally Invasive Applications: Traditional freehand techniques for pedicle screw insertion require direct visualization of bony anatomy and pedicle screw starting points. As technologies have evolved to include 3D navigation and robotics, they have allowed for reliable placement of pedicle screws in a more minimally invasive manner requiring less surgical dissection. Rather than a direct open exposure, pedicles are accessed via percutaneous or transmuscular approaches.

MIS (minimally invasive surgery) approaches using robotics for adult spinal deformity including anterior, lateral, and posterior techniques have been reported with similar outcomes to open procedures.[31–33] Many of these methods can be used to correct coronal deformity and sagittal balance at lower lumbar levels. Similar techniques may be useful in specific types of scoliotic curves in pediatric patients; however, current evidence is lacking and further investigation is needed.

Limitations

The use of CT-guided navigation and robotics is not without its limitations. In addition to increased radiation to the patient as discussed previously, there are concerns regarding cost and operative workflow. Because health-care costs have continued to increase during the past few years, there is an increased emphasis on reducing them in today's environment. Three-dimensional navigation and robotic systems have a large up-front cost often exceeding US$1 million but can theoretically lead to cost-savings to the system over time through improved patient outcomes and decreased numbers of reoperations. As stated previously, Baky and colleagues[19] found that in pediatric scoliosis patients undergoing fusion, no patients in whom navigation was used required a return to the OR for malpositioned screws, as compared with 3.6% in the fluoroscopic guidance group. Revision spine surgery is expensive,[34] thus eliminating this need in even a small sum of patients by using navigation could have a large impact. However, most studies investigation operative time when using navigation and robotics have found no difference or an increase in the navigation group.[17–19] Thus, increased OR time is another potential added cost associated with navigation but as surgeons and OR staff become more comfortable with the technology, the setup and workflow time will hopefully improve. To date, there are no studies directly comparing cost-effectiveness of these new technologies to traditional freehand or fluoroscopic techniques.

An area of interest regarding machine vision technology specifically is the potential for decreased image acquisition time, which helps improve operating room (OR) workflow, especially if additional registrations are required.

Compared with traditional fluoroscopic navigation, which requires repositioning the machine at the desired level and completing a full spin for a new registration, machine vision navigation has a rapid reregistration system that takes less than 30 seconds. This is because a reregistration can be performed by simply readjusting the camera followed by a visible light projection and digitization for 3D-image reconstruction. Malham and colleagues[25] reported an initial registration time in their study of 106 seconds and rapid reregistration if needed, took an average of 22.7 seconds. Similarly, Jakubovic and colleagues[35] found a significant improvement in registration workflow with machine vision versus traditional navigation systems (41 vs 258–794 seconds; $P < .05$).

Navigation must be used with caution and a high index of suspicion that the frame of reference on the reconstructed images corresponds precisely to the direct anatomy encountered during cases. The potential for inaccurate registration is a concern for patient safety and requires conversion to traditional freehand or fluoroscopic techniques in some cases.[17] This concern is amplified as the working level increases in distance from the reference array. Navigation systems use a dynamic reference array attached to the patient in order to enable tool tracking. Increasing working distance from this array can lead to inaccuracies. Guha and colleagues[36] performed a cadaveric study to quantify this. They found an increase in navigation error of greater than 2 mm at greater than 2 levels from the reference array due to surgical manipulation and respiratory induced motion. This is concerning particularly in pediatric scoliosis cases with more levels included in the fusion construct because they could require multiple reregistrations to remain accurate.

SUMMARY

Current technologies for image guidance navigation and robotic assistance with spinal surgery are improving rapidly with several systems commercially available. Purported advantages of these systems include increased accuracy of pedicle screw placement, decreased surgeon radiation exposure, and potential for minimally invasive applications. There is also potential for increased pedicle screw density in long fusion constructs due to navigation allowing for the placement of screws at difficult levels where hooks or wires would have been necessary to safely obtain fixation previously. Limitations regarding cost, workflow issues, and inaccurate registrations remain, although hopefully these are mitigated as surgeons and OR teams become more familiar with the technology. Newer machine vision technology has several potential advantages. Limited studies have shown similar outcomes to traditional navigation platforms with decreased intraoperative radiation and time required for registration. However, there are no active robotic arms that can be coupled with machine vision navigation. Further research is necessary to justify the cost, potential increased operative time and workflow issues but the use of navigation and robotics will only continue to expand given the growing body of evidence supporting their use.

DISCLOSURE

The authors have no commercial or financial conflicts of interest or funding sources to report.

REFERENCES

1. Karkenny AJ, Mendelis JR, Geller DS, et al. The role of intraoperative navigation in orthopaedic surgery. J Am Acad Orthop Surg 2019;27(19):e849–58.
2. Kochanski RB, Lombardi JM, Laratta JL, et al. Image-guided navigation and robotics in spine surgery. Neurosurgery 2019;84(6):1179–89.
3. Horsley VCR. The structure and functions of the cerebellum examined by a new method. Brain 1908;31:45–124.
4. Kalfas IH, Kormos DW, Murphy MA, et al. Application of frameless stereotaxy to pedicle screw fixation of the spine. J Neurosurg 1995;83(4):641–7.
5. Saragaglia D, Picard F, Leitner F. An 8- to 10-year follow-up of 26 computer-assisted total knee arthroplasties. Orthopedics 2007;30(10 Suppl):S121–3.
6. Malham GM, Wells-Quinn T. What should my hospital buy next?-Guidelines for the acquisition and application of imaging, navigation, and robotics for spine surgery. J Spine Surg 2019;5(1):155–65.
7. Chung KJ, Suh SW, Desai S, et al. Ideal entry point for the thoracic pedicle screw during the free hand technique. Int Orthop 2008;32(5):657–62.
8. Parker SL, McGirt MJ, Farber SH, et al. Accuracy of free-hand pedicle screws in the thoracic and lumbar spine: analysis of 6816 consecutive screws. Neurosurgery 2011;68(1):170–8 [discussion: 178].
9. Modi H, Suh SW, Song HR, et al. Accuracy of thoracic pedicle screw placement in scoliosis using the ideal pedicle entry point during the freehand technique. Int Orthop 2009;33(2):469–75.
10. Lonstein JE, Denis F, Perra JH, et al. Complications associated with pedicle screws. J Bone Joint Surg Am 1999;81(11):1519–28.
11. Suk SI, Kim WJ, Lee SM, et al. Thoracic pedicle screw fixation in spinal deformities: are they really safe? Spine (Phila Pa 1976) 2001;26(18):2049–57.
12. Kim YJ, Lenke LG, Bridwell KH, et al. Free hand pedicle screw placement in the thoracic spine: is it safe? Spine (Phila Pa 1976) 2004;29(3):333–42 [discussion: 342].
13. Laine T, Makitalo K, Schlenzka D, et al. Accuracy of pedicle screw insertion: a prospective CT study in 30 low back patients. Eur Spine J 1997;6(6):402–5.
14. Laine T, Lund T, Ylikoski M, et al. Accuracy of pedicle screw insertion with and without computer assistance: a randomised controlled clinical study in 100 consecutive patients. Eur Spine J 2000;9(3):235–40.
15. Van de Kelft E, Costa F, Van der Planken D, et al. A prospective multicenter registry on the accuracy of pedicle screw placement in the thoracic, lumbar, and sacral levels with the use of the O-arm imaging system and StealthStation Navigation. Spine (Phila Pa 1976) 2012;37(25):E1580–7.
16. Molliqaj G, Schatlo B, Alaid A, et al. Accuracy of robot-guided versus freehand fluoroscopy-assisted pedicle screw insertion in thoracolumbar spinal surgery. Neurosurg Focus 2017;42(5):E14.
17. Ringel F, Stuer C, Reinke A, et al. Accuracy of robot-assisted placement of lumbar and sacral pedicle screws: a prospective randomized comparison to conventional freehand screw implantation. Spine (Phila Pa 1976) 2012;37(8):E496–501.
18. Baldwin KD, Kadiyala M, Talwar D, et al. Does intraoperative CT navigation increase the accuracy of pedicle screw placement in pediatric spinal deformity surgery? A systematic review and meta-analysis. Spine Deform 2022;10(1):19–29.
19. Baky FJ, Milbrandt T, Echternacht S, et al. Intraoperative computed tomography-guided navigation for pediatric spine patients reduced return to operating room for screw malposition compared with freehand/fluoroscopic techniques. Spine Deform 2019;7(4):577–81.
20. Gonzalez D, Ghessese S, Cook D, et al. Initial intraoperative experience with robotic-assisted pedicle screw placement with stealth navigation in pediatric spine deformity: an evaluation of the first 40 cases. J Robot Surg 2021;15(5):687–93.
21. Ranade A, Samdani AF, Williams R, et al. Feasibility and accuracy of pedicle screws in children younger than eight years of age. Spine (Phila Pa 1976) 2009;34(26):2907–11.
22. Luo TD, Polly DW Jr, Ledonio CG, et al. Accuracy of pedicle screw placement in children 10 years or younger using navigation and intraoperative CT. Clin Spine Surg 2016;29(3):E135–8.
23. Edstrom E, Burstrom G, Persson O, et al. Does augmented reality navigation increase pedicle screw density compared to free-hand technique

in deformity surgery? Single surgeon case series of 44 patients. Spine (Phila Pa 1976) 2020;45(17): E1085–90.

24. Dorilio J, Utah N, Dowe C, et al. Comparing the efficacy of radiation free machine-vision image-guided surgery with traditional 2-dimensional fluoroscopy: a randomized, single-center study. HSS J 2021;17(3):274–80.

25. Malham GM, Munday NR. Comparison of novel machine vision spinal image guidance system with existing 3D fluoroscopy-based navigation system: a randomized prospective study. Spine J 2022; 22(4):561–9.

26. Mendelsohn D, Strelzow J, Dea N, et al. Patient and surgeon radiation exposure during spinal instrumentation using intraoperative computed tomography-based navigation. Spine J 2016;16(3): 343–54.

27. Shrimpton PC, Jansen JT, Harrison JD. Updated estimates of typical effective doses for common CT examinations in the UK following the 2011 national review. Br J Radiol 2016;89(1057): 20150346.

28. Kapoor S, O'Dowd K, Hilis A, et al. The Nottingham radiation protocol for O-arm navigation in paediatric deformity patients: a feasibility study. Eur Spine J 2021;30(7):1920–7.

29. Su AW, McIntosh AL, Schueler BA, et al. How does patient radiation exposure compare with low-dose o-arm versus fluoroscopy for pedicle screw placement in idiopathic scoliosis? J Pediatr Orthop 2017;37(3):171–7.

30. Dabaghi Richerand A, Christodoulou E, Li Y, et al. Comparison of effective dose of radiation during pedicle screw placement using intraoperative computed tomography navigation versus fluoroscopy in children with spinal deformities. J Pediatr Orthop 2016;36(5):530–3.

31. Chou D, Mummaneni P, Anand N, et al. Treatment of the fractional curve of adult scoliosis with circumferential minimally invasive surgery versus traditional, open surgery: an analysis of surgical outcomes. Glob Spine J 2018;8(8):827–33.

32. Anand N, Baron EM, Khandehroo B, et al. Long-term 2- to 5-year clinical and functional outcomes of minimally invasive surgery for adult scoliosis. Spine (Phila Pa 1976) 2013;38(18):1566–75.

33. Wewel JT, Godzik J, Uribe JS. The utilization of minimally invasive surgery techniques for the treatment of spinal deformity. J Spine Surg 2019; 5(Suppl 1):S84–90.

34. Raman T, Nayar SK, Liu S, et al. Cost-effectiveness of primary and revision surgery for adult spinal deformity. Spine (Phila Pa 1976) 2018;43(11):791–7.

35. Jakubovic R, Guha D, Gupta S, et al. High speed, high density intraoperative 3D optical topographical imaging with efficient registration to MRI and CT for craniospinal surgical navigation. Sci Rep 2018;8(1):14894.

36. Guha D, Jakubovic R, Gupta S, et al. Intraoperative error propagation in 3-dimensional spinal navigation from nonsegmental registration: a prospective cadaveric and clinical study. Glob Spine J 2019;9(5): 512–20.

Shoulder and Elbow

Emerging Technologies in Shoulder Arthroplasty
Navigation, Mixed Reality, and Preoperative Planning

Brenton R. Jennewine, MD[a,b], Tyler J. Brolin, MD[a,c],*

KEYWORDS

- Shoulder arthroplasty • Navigation • Augmented reality • Mixed reality
- Computer-assisted surgery • Patient-specific instrumentation • Preoperative planning

---

KEY POINTS

- Accurate and precise placement of shoulder arthroplasty components is thought to maximize postoperative function and increase long-term implant survival.
- Preoperative planning with 3-dimensional computed tomography scapula reconstructions adds critical information for understanding complex glenoid deformities and being adequately prepared for intraoperative success.
- Patient-specific instrumentation, intraoperative navigation, and mixed reality increase a surgeon's ability to replicate preoperative plans, minimize component malposition, and maximize fixation during shoulder arthroplasty.

INTRODUCTION

With an advancing population age, anatomic and reverse shoulder arthroplasty (aTSA and rTSA, respectively) have a well-established track record in decreasing pain, enhancing patient function, and improving quality of life for the management of end-stage osteoarthritis, irreparable rotator cuff tears, proximal humerus fractures, and rotator cuff arthropathy.[1–3] Both implants have shown excellent long-term survivorship, with 10-year primary aTSA survival rate of 96%[4] and primary rTSA survival rate of 91%[5]; however, complications occur in roughly 11% of aTSA[6] and 16.5% of rTSA procedures.[5] Instability and component loosening, especially the glenoid component, are common complications and causes for revision surgery, with glenoid loosening occurring in 1.2% of rTSAs (7.2% of all rTSA complications) and 3.9% of aTSAs (37.7% of all aTSA complications).[6–9] Glenoid malpositioning represents a factor for these complications.[10–12]

Although the ideal positions for both the humeral and glenoid components are unknown and remain a topic for debate, glenoid positioning in more than 10° to 15° of retroversion leads to more micromotion at the bone-cement surface for aTSA, increased glenoid contact pressures, and significantly increased osteolysis around the central peg in aTSA.[10–12] With regards to rTSA, glenoid fixation is enhanced by maximizing the bone-metal interface, maximizing screw length, and minimizing cortical perforations.[13,14] Guide-pin placement after glenoid exposure remains a critical step for establishing version and inclination, while placing the component on an axis to achieve strong screw purchase in the scapular pillars.[15,16] Re-establishing neutral inclination has been a focus

---

[a] Department of Orthopaedic Surgery and Biomedical Engineering, University of Tennessee Health Science Center-Campbell Clinic, 920 Madison Avenue, Memphis, TN 38163, USA; [b] Campbell Clinic Orthopaedics, 1211 Union Avenue #500, Memphis, TN 38104, USA; [c] Campbell Clinic Orthopaedics, 1400 South Germantown Road, Germantown, TN 38138, USA
* Corresponding author.
E-mail address: tbrolin@campbellclinic.com

Orthop Clin N Am 54 (2023) 209–225
https://doi.org/10.1016/j.ocl.2022.11.006
0030-5898/23/© 2022 Elsevier Inc. All rights reserved.

for placement of the rTSA baseplate given the increase in stress seen at the bone implant interface in biomechanical testing.[17]

Additionally, erroneous screw trajectories in rTSA glenoid baseplate fixation may increase micromotion at the baseplate-bone interface, decreasing bone in-growth, and predisposing to aseptic baseplate loosening,[18] while screw perforation of the glenoid vault is associated with injury to periscapular neurovascular structures and scapular spine fractures.[19–23] To limit baseplate micromotion, biomechanical studies emphasize the importance of accurate screw trajectory,[24] maximizing screw length, especially in the anterior and inferior baseplate screw holes,[25] and using enough screws (between two and four) to achieve stable fixation without decreasing the quality of bone for possible future revisions or increasing the risk of cortical violation.[25,26]

With more than 70% of all shoulder arthroplasty procedures in the United States being completed by surgeons performing fewer than 10 per year, this lower surgical volume and experience could alter component position accuracy and reduce outcomes.[27,28] Additionally, higher degrees of preoperative glenoid deformity and an intraoperative inability to visualize the scapular plane to correctly judge glenoid orientation likely also contribute to the variability and malpositioning of the glenoid components and baseplate screws.[29,30]

The field of shoulder arthroplasty has been investigating various methods to help the surgeon better understand the preoperative deformity, plan for component placement, and execute the surgical plan accurately. The most critical advances so far include preoperative planning with 3-dimensional computed tomography (CT) scapular reconstructions, patient-specific instrumentation (PSI), intraoperative navigation, and intraoperative mixed reality (MR) devices. Debate exists which of these technologies will emerge as the gold standard, and it is prudent for shoulder surgeons to be knowledgeable with all existing technology. The following sections highlight the key features and relevant literature related to these advancements in shoulder arthroplasty.

PREOPERATIVE PLANNING

Background

Preoperative planning is becoming an increasingly studied and utilized trend in order to better understand glenohumeral parameters and accurately execute a shoulder arthroplasty. Although this trend is relatively new in shoulder arthroplasty, the concepts of preoperative planning and implant templating are well established for other orthopedic procedures, especially total knee and hip arthroplasties.[31–33] These plans can help the surgeon better understand patient anatomical considerations and have appropriate implants ready for use; additionally, they may lead to improved surgical outcomes. With this in mind, preoperative planning can play an integral role in achieving better results and implant positioning within shoulder arthroplasties.

Preoperative Imaging–Radiographic to 3-Dimensional

Overview of imaging options

Shoulder arthroplasty preoperative imaging begins with standard shoulder radiographs (ie, Grashey view true-AP, scapular Y, and axillary lateral). The axillary lateral view can provide a general sense of the patient's glenoid version, as well as his or her anteroposterior wear and subluxation patterns, which are critical to evaluate for possible intraoperative correction or augmentation during shoulder arthroplasty. True-AP radiographs can provide knowledge regarding inclination and superior wear typical in later stages of rotator cuff tear arthropathy. Advanced imaging, including MRI and/or 2-dimensional CT, are ordered at the prerogative of the surgeon depending on the concern for rotator cuff pathology or better evaluation of glenoid version, deformity, and available bone stock. Lowe and colleagues[34] investigated glenoid version measurement, Walch classification, and interobserver agreement between CT and MRI, finding MRI and CT have excellent interobserver agreement in calculating the glenoid version and Walch classification for less severe glenoid deformity, but CT may be more suitable to distinguish between type B2 and C glenoids.

With more advanced software and computing capabilities, 3-dimensional CT reconstructions of the scapula and humerus allow for finer-detail analysis of the boney architecture prior to surgery. Several companies have software that can reconstruct 2-dimensional CT into 3-dimensional images along the scapular plane identified by the inferior scapular angle, the scapular trigonum, and the center of the glenoid. Table 1 illustrates commercially available 3-dimensional planning and patient-specific instrumentation systems. From these 3-dimensional CT scans, the glenoid vault model could be used to estimate a patient's normal, premorbid glenoid for use in calculating version and inclination.[35] Fig. 1 shows representative images of the preoperative planning process using Arthrex VIP planning software before rTSA.

Table 1
Available 3-dimensional glenoid planning software and patient-specific instrumentation

Company	System	Reusable PSI?	Description
DJO Global	Match Point System	No	Preoperative 3-dimensional planning system allows for surgeon input on glenoid position. The PSI 3-dimensional guide is manufactured by Materalise for guide pin placement.
Depuy Synthes	TRUMATCH	No	Preoperative 3-dimensional planning system allows for surgeon input on glenoid position. The PSI 3-dimensional guide is manufactured by Materalise for guide pin placement
Zimmer Biomet	Signature ONE	No	Preoperative 3-dimensional planning system allows for surgeon input on glenoid position. Multiple 3-dimensional guides are manufactured for guide pin placement, reaming depth, baseplate impacting, and baseplate screw guide.
Arthrex	OrthoVis and VIP	Yes	Preoperative 3-dimensional planning system allows for surgeon input on glenoid position. Intraoperatively the Arthrex 5-dimensional targeter legs are adjusted to fit the glenoid for planned guide pin trajectory. This is a reusable PSI.
Stryker	Blueprint	No	Preoperative 3-dimensional planning system allows for surgeon input on glenoid position. The PSI 3-dimensional guide is manufactured by Materalise for guide pin placement. Blueprint originally created by Tornier and utilized Glenosys planning software (Imascap). This product was later acquired by Wright Medical and subsequently by Stryker.
Exactech	Equinoxe Planning App	N/A	Preoperative 3-dimensional planning system allows for surgeon input on glenoid position. There is no PSI available, but planning can be used with ExactechGPS navigation system.
Medacta	MyShoulder	No	Preoperative 3-dimensional planning system allows for surgeon input on glenoid position. In-house manufacturing of PSI for guide pin placement and humeral neck cut.

Comparison of 2-dimensional and 3-dimensional computed tomography imaging for glenoid pathology

Axial 2-dimensional CT images are typically used to assess glenoid wear patterns, Walch classification,[16] and version via the method proposed by Friedman and colleagues,[36] while coronal images can assess inclination.[37] However, these measurements made on 2-dimensional imaging are imprecise to accurately depict glenoid deformity. Scalise and colleagues[38] investigated the interobserver reliability for accurate glenoid version, inclination, and area of bone loss between 2-dimensional and 3-dimensional images analyzed by 4 surgeons, finding that 3-dimensional reconstructions allowed for more accurate understanding and better agreement on areas of bone loss that directly affected their proposed implant placement. Kwon and colleagues[39] measured glenoid morphology on 3-dimensional images of cadaveric shoulders, finding a high degree of accuracy compared with their true anatomic measurements. The difference between 2-dimensional and 3-dimensional measurements relates to the plane of image acquisition (gantry angle) for CT scans and the resting scapular rotation, which can vary between patients. Two separate studies showed that small variations in the scapular rotation resulted in significant alterations in version and inclination measurements on 2-dimensional CT scans that are not reformatted in the scapular plane.[40,41] Thus, 3-dimensional reconstructions reduce the variability between CT scanners and

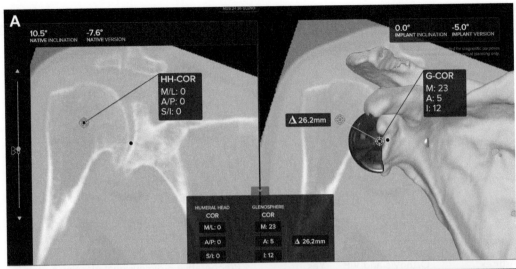

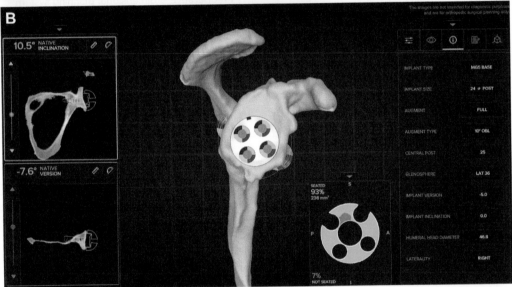

Fig. 1. Representative images of the Arthrex VIP preoperative planning system for rTSA. Part A (*upper*) shows the change in center of rotation between the native humeral head and the proposed placement of the glenosphere. Part B (*lower*) depicts proposed baseplate position on the glenoid indicating native and implant parameters regarding version and inclination.

technicians, which could directly affect glenoid measurements.

As discussed earlier, there are multiple commercially available 3-dimensional planning software systems that calculate glenoid version, inclination, and humeral head subluxation. Various studies have investigated the measurement agreement between these systems and with surgeon measurements, as the systems vary in their method for calculating the previously mentioned values. For instance, Bluprint (Stryker) utilizes an automated process via a best-fit sphere, while several other companies use a manual-input landmark system for

calculation (VIP [Arthrex], Materialise [DJO], and GPS [Exactech]). Denard and colleagues[42] compared glenoid version and inclination measured on 63 patients calculated with Blueprint (Stryker) and VIP (Arthrex) 3-dimensional software. With regards to version and inclination, Blueprint and VIP had agreement within 5° in 69.8% and 54.0% of shoulders, respectively, while more than 10° of variation was seen in 11.1% and 19.0% of shoulders, respectively.[42] This considerable variability was further investigated by Erickson and colleagues,[43] comparing surgeon-calculated 2-dimensional preoperative measurements and those calculated with 4 commonly available 3-dimensional planning systems (Blueprint, VIP, Materialise, and GPS). With surgeon measurements as the reference, Blueprint had less agreement within 5° for version and inclination and more measurements with a greater than 10° difference compared with VIP, Materialise, and GPS. The authors noted that the difference in agreement likely relates to the automated system utilized with Blueprint and the manual method with the other 3 software systems.[43]

3-dimensional reconstructions and their effect on glenoid surgical plans

Glenoid wear patterns can be corrected via 3 main methods: eccentric reaming, bone grafting, or glenoid augmentation. Eccentric reaming remains a viable option for less severe version correction, with eccentric reaming to correct more than 15° of retroversion to neutral is associated with a higher risk of glenoid vault violation.[44,45] Bone grafting larger defects is an effective solution for both aTSA and rTSA, but has a risk for nonunion and resorption that can be alleviated by the use of posterior augmentation to replace grafting.[46,47]

Beyond the more accurate representation of glenoid pathology with 3-dimensional CT scans, these images can be utilized to affect intraoperative decisions. Rosenthal and colleagues[48] investigated how preoperative planning with 2-dimensional versus 3-dimensional imaging affected glenoid version correction methods in patients undergoing a shoulder arthroplasty, finding that surgeons who preoperatively planned with 3-dimensional images chose to use augmented glenoids for version correction in 54% of cases compared with just 15% of cases utilizing 2-dimensional preoperative planning, with the remainder of patients undergoing eccentric reaming for version correction.

Intraoperative glenoid guide-pin placement utilizing 3-dimensional preoperative planning

As previously discussed, accurate glenoid guide-pin placement is a critical step in determining the version, inclination, and final placement of the glenoid component. Free-hand guide-pin placement based on 2-dimensional preoperative imaging can result in high variability in final component position. Jacquot and colleagues[49] utilized the Glenosys 3-dimensional preoperative planning system to find an optimal guide-pin location while utilizing a free-hand technique to place the guide pin. They showed that preoperative planning with 3-dimensional software resulted in high accuracy between preoperative plans and

postoperative guide pin location with mean errors of less than 5° for version and inclination, while having high precision and eliminating outliers causing malposition of the implant based on Throckmorton and colleagues'[50] criteria. Jacquot's group did notice that the freehand technique resulted in the mean guide pin start point being 3 mm from the preoperative plan, with 41% of cases being malpositioned greater than 4 mm, which could lead to baseplate overhang or impingement, an error that was eliminated by the use of patient-specific instrumentation. The high accuracy obtained for guide-pin and glenoid component position utilizing 3-dimensional preoperative planning was further supported by Berhout and colleagues.[51,52]

Preoperative templating

Preoperative templating for component size and position is a critical portion of total joint procedures that has not translated as widely into shoulder arthroplasty. With hip and knee arthroplasties, templating relies on radiographs, with limited use of CT images to assist in the planning process. The converse is likely the case for shoulder arthroplasty. Lee and colleagues[53] utilized calibrated Grashey-view radiographs to template their Tornier Aequalis humerus implant. This group found low inter-rater agreement on templated implant size except for humeral head size, and only 62% of patients received humerus head sizes within 1 size of the preoperative template, with inter-rater preoperative templating agreement and actual implant used even lower for neck angle and stem size. The group remarked that templating from an anteroposterior (AP) radiograph alone is not helpful, as the sagittal plane of the humerus is typically narrower and can greatly affect implant size used in surgery. As an alternative to radiographs, Freehill and colleagues[54] utilized 3-dimensional CT images of the humerus and scapula for templating. They found that final glenoid selection matched preoperative planning perfectly for 89% of cases and within 1 glenoid size for 99% of cases, while a similar agreement was found for both stemmed and stemless humeral components. Freehill concluded that 3-dimensional CT images were a viable imaging option for preoperative templating.

Advances in proximal humerus preoperative planning

Accurate anatomic neck osteotomies in shoulder arthroplasty are necessary for establishing humeral head inclination and retroversion. Understanding the patient's premorbid proximal humerus anatomy is critical, especially in cases of severe osteoarthritis or proximal humerus fractures that make it difficult to determine humeral head height, neck angle, and retroversion. Poltaretskyi and colleagues[55] created and validated a statistical shape model (SSM) that is able to accurately recreate premorbid proximal humerus anatomy for osteoarthritis and proximal humerus fractures with varying diaphyseal extension. Although literature regarding humerus neck cuts is limited, Poltaretskyi's group envisions this SSM being applied to preoperatively plan a neck cut in 3 dimensions and create a patient-specific guide or project the premorbid anatomy onto the patient intraoperatively using augmented reality.

Patient-Specific Instrumentation
Background
Patient-specific instrumentation (PSI) is not a novel technique within orthopedics and has been utilized in other fields including total hip and knee arthroplasties.[56] Within the field of shoulder arthroplasty, PSI refers to sterilizable instruments that have been created based on preoperative 3-dimensional planning to better facilitate correct positioning of the components, most commonly the guide pin placement in the glenoid. PSI is an alternative to intraoperative navigation systems, which are expensive, not readily available to most surgeons performing shoulder arthroplasties,[27] have a higher learning curve, and can be cumbersome to use. PSI may provide similar levels of accuracy as navigation, while reducing the surgical cost and steps associated with navigation.

Importantly, PSI relies on 3-dimensional CT images and requires user input for the creation of the ideal guide pin trajectory, applying much of the same principles and outcomes discussed previously in preoperative imaging. Most commercial shoulder arthroplasty companies offer 3-dimensional planning software that is integrated with a manufacturing side to create these instruments with a typical turnaround of 3 to 6 weeks. The glenoid guide is typically 3-dimensionally printed using sterilizable resin that will sit on the patient's glenoid intraoperatively with a drill hole aligning the preplanned trajectory.[57,58] Some companies allow for the use of reusable glenoid targeting guides that can minimize the cost associated with PSI implementation (eg, the Arthrex 5D glenoid targeter guide).

Application and outcomes for patient-specific instrumentation
Several studies have showed greatly increased accuracy with PSI based on 3-dimensional preoperative planning. Hendel and colleagues[59] performed a prospective randomized controlled trial investigating the accuracy of 3-dimensional planning with the PSI method or 2-dimensional planning with a free-hand guide-pin placement intraoperatively to place a glenoid in neutral version and inclination. This group showed the use of 3-dimensional imaging and PSI is more accurate and precise, especially with regards to inclination and preoperative retroversion greater than 16° as the mean deviation from neutral version was retroverted 1.2° with PSI and retroverted 10° with conventional planning and instrumentation.[59] This was similarly supported by Throckmorton and colleagues,[50] who compared PSI and traditional instrumentation for aTSA and rTSA glenoid components, finding PSI guides to be more accurate and greatly reduce the amount of significant malpositioned components. Considered a landmark study applying 3-dimensional planning and PSI, Iannotti and colleagues[60] investigated glenoid guide-pin accuracy with standard instrumentation using 2-dimensional CT planning, 3-dimensional CT planning alone, and 3-dimensional CT planning with PSI. In this study, OrthoVis 3-dimensional software was used for glenoid component planning (neutral version and inclination) and to create a printed 3-dimensional model of the glenoid architecture with planned guide-pin placement for the PSI group. Intraoperatively, the Glenoid Intelligent Reusable Instrument System (Custom Orthopedic Solutions; now the Arthrex 5-dimensional glenoid targeter guide) was placed over the sterilized model's guide pin, and the guide's tines were adjusted to fit over the model's rim, customizing the PSI to the patient's anatomy for guide-pin placement. The authors found no significant difference in version, inclination, or entry point for 3-dimensional planned glenoid with or without the PSI, but did find that either 3-dimensional system (with or without the PSI) resulted in significant improvements in accuracy compared to 2-dimensional planning with standard instrumentation for guide-pin placement.[60] Fig. 2 shows intraoperative use of the Arthrex 5-dimensional targeter guide for guide-pin placement.

A systematic review and meta-analysis on PSI versus standard instrumentation published by Cabarcas and colleagues[61] found that standard instrumentation resulted in mean errors of 7.1° (range 3.5°–11.2°) for version, 8.45° (range 2.8°–11.65°) for inclination, and 2.6 mm (range 1.7–3.4 mm) for entry point offset. With the use of PSI, the average mean errors were reduced

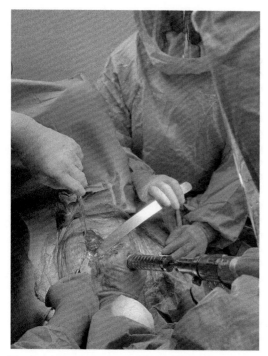

Fig. 2. Intraoperative use of the Arthrex 5-dimensional targeter guide for glenoid guide-pin placement.

to 3.47° (range 0.5°–4.49°) for version, 2.36° (range 0.1°–4°) for inclination, and 1.67 mm (range 1.09–2.4 mm) for entry point offset.[61]

Villatte and colleagues[62] published a meta-analysis including 7 clinical and 5 cadaveric studies comparing 3-dimensional planned PSI with standard instrumentation, finding that while PSI provided higher accuracy, the mean difference between PSI (version: 2.73° ± 0.48; inclination: 1.88° ± 0.41; entry point 1.06 mm ± 0.2) and standard instrumentation (version: 5.88° ± 1.10; inclination: 5.78° ± 0.98; entry point 2.04 mm ± 0.4) was small and likely not clinically relevant. However, the percentage of components classified as outliers or significantly malpositioned was 68.6% using standard instruments and 15.3% using PSI, going further to state that PSI was much more accurate and precise, with higher degrees of preoperative retroversion or more complex glenoid deformity.[62] Thus, PSI may be more useful in complex deformity correction or for low-volume surgeons where inexperience may lead to higher malpositioned components.

Manufacturing time for PSI can be between 3 and 6 weeks, and costs can be significant, ranging from $500 to 1200.[58] For this reason, Darwood and colleagues[63] developed and published a novel method to create PSI intraoperatively in a sterile manner in under 4 minutes.

Preoperatively, the group performed standard 3-dimensional planning and uploaded their guide pin planned trajectory into a robot fitted with sterile drapes and a drill in the operating room. After the glenoid is exposed, an elastic membrane blank is filled with a sterile moldable polymer. Once filled, the mold is pressed into the patient's glenoid and allowed to harden, creating a 3-dimensional replica of the surface of the glenoid. This hardened mold is placed on the robot, which utilizes the preoperative 3-dimensional plans to drill a guide for the glenoid pin. Once finished, the patient-specific instrument is ready for use. This group trialed this method on 24 cadaver shoulders and found exceptionally high accuracy with mean variations of guide-pin placement within 2° degrees of preoperatively planned version and inclination.[63] This method or reusable glenoid guide system (Arthrex 5-dimensional targeter) offers a promising solution to manufacturing time and costly commercial PSI.

Limitations

Further limitations do exist with the application of PSI. Gomes and Hendel and colleagues[57,59] both note that the software performing the 3-dimensional reconstruction and PSI creation may or may not remove calcified labrum or osteophytes; thus the PSI would require the surgeon to leave these structures in place until the guide pin is drilled or the PSI will not fit accurately. As adequate exposure of the glenoid can be difficult in patients, PSI use requires perfect exposure of the glenoid to clean off soft tissues that may prevent the guide from seating well. Additionally, most PSI utilizes a single guide-pin placement, which can predispose to off-axis reaming.[59,64] Finally, there are few data relating high accuracy of the guide-pin placement and glenoid component position to clinical outcomes. Also, reaming depth is not typically incorporated into PSI guides, which affects overall medialization of the joint line and is difficult to assess intraoperatively.

Summary Regarding the Use of Preoperative Planning

Preoperative planning with 3-dimensional CT images and the use of patient-specific instrumentation have been shown to improve the accuracy between the individual surgeon's preoperative ideal glenoid or humeral position and the final implanted position. Furthermore, the use of 2-dimensional imaging systems for measuring preoperative inclination and version may be inaccurate, compared with

3-dimensional imaging.[65] There are few data yet that clinically correlate this to improved patient outcomes, namely because of a lack of data that support what the correct glenoid version or inclination should be.[52] Some argue that the glenoid should be placed ideally at neutral version avoiding more than 15° degrees of retroversion and 0°-10° of inferior inclination to decrease stress on the rotator cuff and at the bone-implant surface.[10–12,66] Another school of thought supports recreation of the patient's pre-morbid version and inclination. Additionally, other factors such as glenoid guide pin entry point and reaming depth may also be critical for correct glenoid placement.[52] Future investigations are needed to elucidate what the ideal glenoid position should be, as preoperative 3-dimensional planning and patient-specific instrumentation can help achieve this accurately.

NAVIGATION
Background
Intraoperative navigation is a familiar concept within orthopedic surgery, especially within the fields of hip and knee arthroplasty, where its utilization has become more common.[67–69] Evidence within these fields has shown that navigation can improve accurate placement of components, while reducing outliers leading to malpositioning.[69,70] Similarly, navigation could offer great benefits in shoulder arthroplasty, especially with regards to accuracy of the humeral head cut, glenoid component position, and stable fixation of glenoid baseplate for rTSA; however, navigation has not become as utilized for shoulder arthroplasty as it has for knee and hip arthroplasty. As stated previously, proper glenoid position can potentially decrease glenoid loosening and decrease need for revisions, offering advantages similar to patient-specific instrumentation, MR, and 3-dimensional CT preoperative planning. Specific advantages related to navigation include the ability to detect glenoid reaming depth, improve reverse arthroplasty baseplate screw trajectory to maximize length, and offer dynamic real-time feedback. An important utility of navigation is the real-time feedback for ideal trajectory and screw length with glenoid baseplate fixation. As discussed previously, accurate trajectory of baseplate screws is critical to minimize complications and maximize screw purchase to decrease micromotion and aseptic loosening.[18–26]

Many commercial and noncommercial investigational navigation systems exist and are reported in the literature. The typical process for navigation involves preoperative and intraoperative steps that can increase planning and surgical times.[71,72] Preoperatively, either 2-dimensional or 3-dimensional CT scans are uploaded to planning software where the surgeon plans preferred humeral cuts, glenoid component position with or without use of augmentation or grafting, and baseplate screw trajectory for rTSA. After glenoid exposure intraoperatively, a registration process occurs to allow the navigation system to orient the preoperative plan with the patient's anatomy. Registration typically occurs with a fixed optical sensor on the coracoid and manual pinpoint registration of unique points along the acromion, coracoid, and glenoid face. Following registration, most commercial systems utilize optical tracking devices on the drills and saws to achieve correct orientation with planned measurements. The following section reviews important literature regarding the validity, accuracy, and limitations of navigation for shoulder arthroplasty. An overview of the commercially available navigation systems can be found in Table 2.

Intraoperative Navigation for Shoulder Arthroplasty
In one of the earliest studies regarding shoulder arthroplasty navigation, Edwards and colleagues[73] published a validation study for intraoperative navigation, confirming a high degree of agreement between intraoperative measurements made with navigation and postoperative CT measurements. Aminov and colleagues[74] utilized a dental navigation system (Navigate Surgical Technologies) to trial navigation on 3-dimensional printed scapula models to assist with glenoid guide-pin placement with planned neutral version and inclination, finding high accuracy with near-perfect placement of the guide pin. The authors of this study noted the cheap, low-profile, and already wide availability of this navigation system. Nguyen and colleagues[75] compared glenoid implant position in anatomic shoulder replacement using standard instrumentation with navigation using 3-dimensional models of 16 cadaver shoulders with preprocedure 3-dimensional CT planning for neutral glenoid version and inclination. Navigation was significantly more accurate than standard instrumentation for final implant version (1.5° ± 1.9° and 7.4° ± 3.8, respectively), with no significance found for final inclination, but navigation was more accurate. The authors measured version at all steps for glenoid component placement–guide pin, reaming, and final implantation after cementing–finding significant alterations and increased variability in version and inclination

Table 2
Intraoperative shoulder arthroplasty navigation systems

Company	System	Description
Exactech	ExactechGPS	Utilizes a fixed tracker placed into the coracoid, as well as landmark registration. Instruments are tracked during all steps of glenoid component placement: guide pin placement, reaming, baseplate and glenosphere placement, and baseplate screw depth/trajectory. Used with the Exactech Equinoxe shoulder system.
Kinamed	NaviPro Shoulder	Navigation system that can be universally used with all shoulder systems – reverse or anatomic. Tacking system used for glenoid component placement, as well as humeral cut version and inclination measurement.

during the reaming and cementation steps for standard and navigated processed. They noted while guide-pin placement is a critical step for final position, off-axis reaming and nonsymmetric seating during cementation may be other sources of component placement error that would benefit from the navigation process.[76]

Several cadaveric studies using navigation for glenoid guide-pin placement have been published, finding that navigation resulted in high accuracy. Using the ExactechGPS system, Colasanti and colleagues[77] had an average mean guide-pin placement of 3.1° plus or minus 2° in anteversion and inferior inclination of 5.4° when planning for neutral version and 10° of inferior tilt. Verborgt and colleagues[78] performed a cadaveric study on 14 shoulders using 2-dimensional CT planning (neutral version and 10° inferior tilt) to compare glenoid component and baseplate screw placement with and without navigation. Navigation resulted in significantly more accurate component placement than without navigation in both version (3.1° vs 8.7° anteversion, respectively) and inclination (−5.4° vs +0.9°, respectively), with postprocedure dissection finding less glenoid vault screw violation with navigation (2 screws with navigation and 5 without).[78]

Similar to cadaveric studies, multiple studies investigating navigated shoulder arthroplasty in patients have been published. Kircher and colleagues[79] reported on increased surgical time needed for 2-dimensional CT-planned navigation in a small cohort of patients. Because of significant issues and errors with the intraoperative registration process, navigation was aborted in 6 cases, but of those completed, navigation increased surgical time by 31 minutes (169.5 minutes with navigation vs 138 minutes without navigation), which could be explained by a higher learning curve needed with navigation to become efficient, as this study only included 10 patients in the navigation arm.[79] The possible

learning curve associated with navigation was investigated by Wang and colleagues[80] utilizing the ExactechGPS system in 24 reverse arthroplasties. Compared with Kircher and colleagues,[80] Wang's study found little difference in surgical time utilizing navigation (77.3 minutes ± 11.8 with navigation and 78.5 minutes ± 18.1 without navigation), and found that surgical time seemed to decrease and plateau after the first 8 cases of a surgeon utilizing navigation for reverse shoulder arthroplasty. Finally, Schoch and colleagues[81] reported on glenoid component position accuracy with navigation, comparing high-volume attending surgeons with lower-volume orthopedic surgery fellows. Using the ExactechGPS system, the mean errors compared with preoperative plans were reported. The mean version error was 6.4° anteverted, with 49% of shoulders exceeding 5° of error and 25% exceeding 10°. Similarly, the mean inclination error was 6.6° of superior tilt (50% exceeded 5° of error and 25% exceeding 10°), and the mean guide pin entry point error was 3.2 mm, with 18% exceeding 4 mm.[81] With these measurements, navigation resulted in 48% of components being malpositioned based on the criteria from Throckmorton and colleagues.[50] While this is considerable, the authors note that their malpositioning was less with navigation than those with standard instrumentation without navigation seen in Throckmorton's study, recommending the use of navigation or patient-specific instrumentation for lower-volume surgeons.[81]

Sadoghi and colleagues[82] published a systematic review of 5 studies including 117 navigated and 114 non-navigated shoulder anatomic and reverse arthroplasties investigating glenoid component placement accuracy, with the included studies planning for neutral version and 0° tilt of the component. They found navigation resulted in significantly improved accuracy utilizing navigation for version (4.4° ± 0.41 with navigation and 10.6° ± 0.67 without navigation.[82] Similarly, Burns and colleagues[83] performed a review of 9 studies comparing glenoid component placement utilizing PSI or navigation with standard instrumentation. When analyzing studies with control groups (standard instrumentation), both PSI and navigation resulted in significant improvements in accuracy of guide-pin placement compared with standard instrumentation resulting in a higher amount of malpositioned implants.[83] With these results in mind, the authors recommended the use of either PSI or navigation to improve the inaccuracy that occurs with standard instrumentation.

Because of the previously mentioned importance of glenoid baseplate screw fixation, several studies also investigated the effect navigation has on baseplate fixation in rTSA. Moreschini and colleagues[84] compared baseplate screw number to achieve solid fixation and mean length of baseplate screw implanted with ExactechGPS navigation compared to preoperative planning with just 2-dimensional CT imaging. They found that navigation required only 11 more minutes of surgical time and resulted in a mean screw length of 35.5 mm with navigation versus 29.2 mm without navigation, also noting that more than 2 screws were needed for stable fixation in only 40.9% of patients with navigation but 85% of patients without navigation. Similarly, Hones and colleagues[85] performed a similar study with 200 patients divided equally between baseplate screw placement with and without navigation, finding a significant increase in average screw lengths with navigation (35 mm with navigation and 32.6 mm without navigation). Finally, Sprowls and colleagues[86] found that navigation resulted in longer mean screw length (36.7 mm with navigation and 30 mm without navigation), longer composite screw length (84 mm with navigation and 76 mm without navigation), and more baseplates achieving solid fixation with just 2 screws (68.6% with navigation and 50.8% without navigation). This group also noted navigation increased operative times by roughly 13 minutes and significantly improved accuracy of component version.

Although much of the literature regarding navigation in shoulder arthroplasty revolves around the glenoid, there are a few studies looking at navigation for the humeral component. Humeral head osteotomy can dictate the component height, version, and neck-shaft angle (NSA), and alterations in these values can predispose to early failure or complications. For instance, a humeral cut too low can damage the cuff insertion and tuberosities, or increase instability, while a cut too high can potentially overstuff the joint leading to early failure.[1,87,88] To investigate the use of navigation during the humeral neck osteotomy, Cavanagh and colleagues[89] utilized 3-dimensional printed shoulders from cadaver models to compare the use of a PSI with navigation based on preplanned values for the humeral height, version, and NSA. They found that there was no significant or clinically relevant difference between using a PSI jig or navigation for the osteotomy in either arthritic or nonarthritic shoulders.

Summary Regarding Navigated Shoulder Arthroplasty

As in knee and hip arthroplasty, navigation in shoulder arthroplasty can have great benefits on improving the accuracy of the glenoid component position, maximizing baseplate fixation, and decreasing the occurrence of malpositioned implants or baseplate screws. Additionally, similar to PSI, navigation may be more beneficial for lower-volume surgeons to limit implant malpositioning.[81] However, there are a number of limitations, including the added surgical time supported by most studies,[79,84,86] high cost, intraoperative navigation malfunctioning,[79] and lack of easy portability. Compared with PSI, navigation can be used for baseplate screw placement, but the accuracy for glenoid guide-pin placement or humeral neck osteotomy is not significantly different with navigation. More studies are needed to justify the utility of navigation over PSI for use in shoulder arthroplasty, especially in anatomic TSA when baseplate screw fixation is not of concern.

MIXED REALITY
Background

As has been discussed, 3-dimensional preoperative planning, patient-specific instrumentation, and intraoperative navigation can greatly improve surgical plans, produce fewer malpositioned implants, and increase the overall accuracy for glenoid positioning. Despite this, PSI and navigation are expensive. Additionally, PSI product turnaround is slow, navigation can be cumbersome to utilize in the operating room, and both increase surgical or preoperative planning time.[62,82] An alternative or adjunct to the previously mentioned methods of accurate glenoid component placement revolves around the cutting-edge technology of MR (or augmented reality [AR]) devices. MR devices are being introduced into the literature and fields of neurosurgery and vascular surgery, with orthopedic surgery following suit. Within orthopedic surgery, MR has been investigated for the use in education, spine instrumentation, trauma involving pelvic and femur fractures, osteotomies, and hip and knee arthroplasty.[90] An overview of available MR systems in shoulder arthroplasty can be found in Table 3.

Application of Mixed Reality in Shoulder Arthroplasty

Thus far, MR has been mainly limited to 3-dimensional models, cadavers, and in patients to a limited extent, but there is great promise for more widespread application. This is especially true for shoulder arthroplasty for similar reasons to the use of navigation and PSI: glenoid component positioning and better understanding of patient anatomy intraoperatively.

One of the earlier applications of MR technology was published in 2019 by Berhouet and colleagues[91], who utilized a novel method to approximate a patient's premorbid glenoid anatomy and project this onto the surgical field to aid in glenoid component placement. In this study, Berhouet's team created a 3-dimensional CT library of healthy, generic scapula models and devised a method to create a crude premorbid 3-dimensional image of a patient's glenoid and scapula. This crude model was morphed with a similar generic scapula out of their library to create a refined glenoid/scapula model that best approximated the patient's premorbid state. This 3-dimensional reconstruction was uploaded to Epson Moverio BT-200 smart glasses (Seiko Epson Corporation, Nagano, Suwa, Japan), which would be worn by the surgeon to project the premorbid scapula onto the patient's shoulder intraoperatively. This ideally would allow the surgeon to better understand premorbid anatomy for correct glenoid guide-pin placement.[91]

Following this, Kriechling and colleagues[92,93] investigated the use of MR technology on glenoid guide-pin placement in a 3-dimensional printed scapula model, followed by a cadaveric study. This group utilized 3-dimensional CT for preoperative planning of guide-pin placement for rTSA, aiming for 0° version and inclination with an inferiorly oriented entry point for an inferiorly placed baseplate. The plan was uploaded to Microsoft cloud and the Microsoft HoloLens1 (Microsoft Corporation, Redmond, Washington). Kriechling created a custom registration device to pinpoint the acromion, coracoid, and glenoid to match the intraoperative surface with the 3-dimensional CT. After registration, the 3-dimensional scapula image and planned guide pin trajectory are holographically projected onto the surgeon's field of view through the glasses. High accuracy of the guide pin trajectory on postoperative CT was found utilizing the above MR method. The 3-dimensional model method resulted in a mean trajectory error (encompassing version and inclination) of 2.7° plus or minus 1.3 and entry point error of 2.3 mm plus or minus 1.1, while cadaveric use resulted in similarly accurate placement with mean trajectory error of 3.8 plus or minus 1.7 and entry point error of 3.5 mm plus or minus 1.7.[94,95]

In similar studies, Schlueter-Brust and colleagues and Gregory and colleagues utilized Microsoft's HoloLens2 technology without the use of an intraoperative registration

Table 3 Mixed reality systems in shoulder arthroplasty		
Company	**System**	**Description**
Stryker	Blueprint Mixed Reality	Preoperative 3-dimensional planning with Blueprint. Headset worn intraoperatively shows 3-dimensional image of preoperative humeral and glenoid plans.
Microsoft	HoloLens	Preoperative 3-dimensional planning is uploaded to the HoloLens worn intraoperatively. The HoloLens overlays a holographic image of the preoperative plan. Used in several studies with and without a registration process. Registration process can help the holographic image overlay to remain fixed on the patient's anatomy intraoperatively.
Medacta	NextAR	Preoperative 3-dimensional planning with MyShoulder. Intraoperative hybrid navigation and MR system that utilizes a fixed tracker on the coracoid and instrument trackers for all steps of glenoid component placement. NextAR Smart Glasses worn intraoperatively displays the real-time feedback from the navigated system with the preoperative plan.

process.[94,95] Schlueter-Brust's team performed a cadaveric study investigating the accuracy of glenoid guide-pin placement with a preoperatively planned 3-dimensional scapular image overlayed via the MR device without a registration process. Their results showed a mean trajectory error (again accounting for combined inclination and version) of 3.9 plus or minus 2.4 and entry point error of 2.4 mm plus or minus 0.7.[96] Gregory and colleagues[95] performed a reverse shoulder arthroplasty utilizing the HoloLens2 on the patient. Intraoperatively, the HoloLens2 projected the preoperative plan on the patient's unregistered glenoid, while the HoloLens2 was connected to a video conference with 4 other surgeons in different countries who could offer real-time advice and adjust the heads-up display (HUD). Although actual measurements of the glenoid component position were not measured, the authors noted adequate position of the component with a surgical duration of 90 minutes.

In the most recent and advanced use of MR technology, Rojas and colleagues[96] described a procedure to use a combination of MR technology and intraoperative navigation on a patient undergoing rTSA. The 3-dimensional preoperative plans were uploaded to a navigated MR system NextAR (Medacta International), which utilizes an intraoperative control-unit (CU) with video display, a fixed tracking device implanted into the coracoid via K-wire, camera tracker that is attachable to all surgical instruments, and glasses to provide a HUD for the surgeon. Registration begins with the 4 borders of the glenoid and then incorporates 15 unique points on the coracoid and glenoid to overlay the 3-dimensional plan onto both the CU and the surgeon's HUD. During all steps of glenoid component placement (utilizing the variably applied camera tracker), the surgeon is provided with real-time versus planned trajectory information, including version, inclination, entry-point position, reaming depth, baseplate placement, and ideal baseplate screw trajectory to maximize length.[96]

Advantages and Limitations of Mixed Reality Technology

These prior studies each show the various advantages and limitations for the application of MR technology in shoulder arthroplasty. Overall, the accuracy of guide-pin placement using MR technology is better compared to free-hand placement, lending to its great prospect in helping maximize accuracy and decrease malpositioning, especially for lower-volume surgeons.[61,92–94] MR technology provides real-time information of glenoid component placement similar to navigation as opposed to PSI with delayed post-operative feedback. The display of information on the HUD allows the surgeon to stay focused on the surgical field compared with pure navigation strategies, and the tracker registration process is simple to use.[96] Registration simplifies and streamlines the HUD overlay process. Schlueter-Brust and colleagues and Gregory and colleagues note the need to virtually drag, rotate, and resize the overlayed scapular hologram while holding the surgeon's head still to keep the scapula hologram from moving, while registration establishes and maintains the virtual position of the scapular hologram on the patient.[92–96]

Limitations are related to the typical availability of these MR head-sets, preoperative 3-dimensional planning software, cost, and possibility for coracoid fracture if a combined MR-navigation strategy is used.[96] The Microsoft HoloLens2 retails for $3500, which is more expensive than PSI but is reusable and vastly cheaper than navigation systems. Additionally, most available MR wearable devices are designed for entertainment and multimedia viewing, which may hinder the accuracy and precision.[91–95]

Summary and Future Ventures for Mixed Reality in Shoulder Arthroplasty

Mixed or augmented-reality provides an exciting application to the field of shoulder arthroplasty that improves on the possible disadvantages of 3-dimensional planning alone, PSI, and sole use of intraoperative navigation, while outperforming standard instrument free-hand glenoid guide-pin placement. Literature is limited on the use of this technology in shoulder arthroplasty, and future studies could investigate the use on patients to correlate with clinical outcomes. MR technology is being utilized in medical education, and this technology can similarly be applied to resident training within shoulder arthroplasty, intraoperative telementoring or teleconferencing for difficult glenoid deformities or surgeons early into practice, and postoperative performance evaluation and critiquing.[95,97]

SUMMARY

Although the ideal component positions to optimize patient outcomes following shoulder arthroplasty remain unknown, accurate placement of the glenoid and humeral components is critical for long-term survival. Preoperative planning with 3-dimensional CT is becoming a commonly utilized strategy to better understand patient anatomy for operative success. Further research is needed and warranted to find the role of other intraoperative assistive devices in shoulder arthroplasty, including patient-specific instrumentation, navigation, and MR; however, this field is already showing great promise towards achieving this goal and likely represents the future of shoulder arthroplasty.

CLINICS CARE POINTS

- Accurate and precise placement of shoulder arthroplasty components is thought to maximize postoperative function and increase long-term implant survival.
- Preoperative planning with 3-dimensional CT scapula reconstructions adds critical information for understanding complex glenoid deformities and being adequately prepared for intraoperative success.
- Patient-specific instrumentation, intraoperative navigation, and MR increase a surgeon's ability to replicate preoperative plans, minimize component malposition, and maximize fixation during shoulder arthroplasty.

DISCLOSURE

The authors have nothing to disclose.

REFERENCES

1. Iannotti JP, Spencer EE, Winter U, et al. Prosthetic positioning in total shoulder arthroplasty. J Shoulder Elbow Surg 2005;14(1 Suppl S):111S–21S.
2. Singh JA, Sperling J, Buchbinder R, et al. Surgery for shoulder osteoarthritis: a Cochrane systematic review. J Rheumatol 2011;38(4):598–605.
3. Frankle M, Siegal S, Pupello D, et al. The reverse shoulder prosthesis for glenohumeral arthritis associated with severe rotator cuff deficiency. a minimum two-year follow-up study of sixty patients. J Bone Joint Surg Am 2005;87(8):1697–705.
4. Piper C, Neviaser A. Survivorship of anatomic total shoulder arthroplasty. J Am Acad Orthop Surg 2022;30(10):457–65.
5. Chelli M, Boileau P, Domos P, et al. Survivorship of reverse shoulder arthroplasty according to indication, age and gender. J Clin Med 2022;11(10):2677.
6. Bohsali KI, Bois AJ, Wirth MA. Complications of Shoulder Arthroplasty. J Bone Joint Surg Am

2017;99(3):256–69. published correction appears in J Bone Joint Surg Am. 2017 Jun 21;99(12):e67.
7. Boileau P. Complications and revision of reverse total shoulder arthroplasty. Orthop Traumatol Surg Res 2016;102(1 Suppl):S33–43.
8. Fox TJ, Foruria AM, Klika BJ, et al. Radiographic survival in total shoulder arthroplasty. J Shoulder Elbow Surg 2013;22(9):1221–7.
9. Australian Orthopaedic Association National Joint Replacement Registry (AOANJRR). Hip, knee & shoulder arthroplasty annual report, AOA, Adelaide, Available at: https://aoanjrr.sahmri.com/annual-reports-2020. Accessed August 2, 2022.
10. Farron A, Terrier A, Büchler P. Risks of loosening of a prosthetic glenoid implanted in retroversion. J Shoulder Elbow Surg 2006;15(4):521–6.
11. Shapiro TA, McGarry MH, Gupta R, et al. Biomechanical effects of glenoid retroversion in total shoulder arthroplasty. J Shoulder Elbow Surg 2007;16(3 Suppl):S90–5.
12. Ho JC, Sabesan VJ, Iannotti JP. Glenoid component retroversion is associated with osteolysis. J Bone Joint Surg Am 2013;95(12):e82.
13. Chebli C, Huber P, Watling J, et al. Factors affecting fixation of the glenoid component of a reverse total shoulder prothesis. J Shoulder Elbow Surg 2008;17(2):323–7.
14. Nyffeler RW, Werner CM, Gerber C. Biomechanical relevance of glenoid component positioning in the reverse Delta III total shoulder prosthesis. J Shoulder Elbow Surg 2005;14(5):524–8.
15. Karelse A, Kegels L, De Wilde L. The pillars of the scapula. Clin Anat 2007;20(4):392–9.
16. Nerot C, Ohl X. Primary shoulder reverse arthroplasty: surgical technique. Orthop Traumatol Surg Res 2014;100(1 Suppl):S181–90.
17. Gutiérrez S, Walker M, Willis M, et al. Effects of tilt and glenosphere eccentricity on baseplate/bone interface forces in a computational model, validated by a mechanical model, of reverse shoulder arthroplasty. J Shoulder Elbow Surg 2011;20(5):732–9.
18. Bitzer A, Rojas J, Patten IS, et al. Incidence and risk factors for aseptic baseplate loosening of reverse total shoulder arthroplasty. J Shoulder Elbow Surg 2018;27(12):2145–52.
19. Hart ND, Clark JC, Wade Krause FR, et al. Glenoid screw position in the Encore reverse shoulder prosthesis: an anatomic dissection study of screw relationship to surrounding structures. J Shoulder Elbow Surg 2013;22(6):814–20.
20. Leschinger T, Hackl M, Buess E, et al. The risk of suprascapular and axillary nerve injury in reverse total shoulder arthroplasty: an anatomic study. Injury 2017;48(10):2042–9.
21. Molony DC, Cassar Gheiti AJ, Kennedy J, et al. A cadaveric model for suprascapular nerve injury during glenoid component screw insertion in

reverse-geometry shoulder arthroplasty. J Shoulder Elbow Surg 2011;20(8):1323–7.

22. Crosby LA, Hamilton A, Twiss T. Scapula fractures after reverse total shoulder arthroplasty: classification and treatment. Clin Orthop Relat Res 2011; 469(9):2544–9.

23. Otto RJ, Virani NA, Levy JC, et al. Scapular fractures after reverse shoulder arthroplasty: evaluation of risk factors and the reliability of a proposed classification. J Shoulder Elbow Surg 2013;22(11):1514–21.

24. Codsi MJ, Iannotti JP. The effect of screw position on the initial fixation of a reverse total shoulder prosthesis in a glenoid with a cavitary bone defect. J Shoulder Elbow Surg 2008;17(3):479–86.

25. Roche C, DiGeorgio C, Yegres J, et al. Impact of screw length and screw quantity on reverse total shoulder arthroplasty glenoid fixation for 2 different sizes of glenoid baseplates. JSES Open Access 2019;3(4):296–303.

26. James J, Allison MA, Werner FW, et al. Reverse shoulder arthroplasty glenoid fixation: is there a benefit in using four instead of two screws? J Shoulder Elbow Surg 2013;22(8):1030–6.

27. Jain N, Pietrobon R, Hocker S, et al. The relationship between surgeon and hospital volume and outcomes for shoulder arthroplasty. J Bone Joint Surg Am 2004;86(3):496–505.

28. Singh A, Yian EH, Dillon MT, et al. The effect of surgeon and hospital volume on shoulder arthroplasty perioperative quality metrics. J Shoulder Elbow Surg 2014;23(8):1187–94.

29. Papadonikolakis A, Neradilek MB, Matsen FA 3rd. Failure of the glenoid component in anatomic total shoulder arthroplasty: a systematic review of the English-language literature between 2006 and 2012. J Bone Joint Surg Am 2013;95(24):2205–12.

30. Iannotti JP, Greeson C, Downing D, et al. Effect of glenoid deformity on glenoid component placement in primary shoulder arthroplasty. J Shoulder Elbow Surg 2012;21(1):48–55.

31. Tanzer M, Makhdom AM. Preoperative planning in primary total knee arthroplasty. J Am Acad Orthop Surg 2016;24(4):220–30. https://doi.org/10.5435/JAAOS-D-14-00332.

32. Della Valle AG, Padgett DE, Salvati EA. Preoperative planning for primary total hip arthroplasty. J Am Acad Orthop Surg 2005;13(7):455–62.

33. Atesok K, Galos D, Jazrawi LM, et al. Preoperative planning in orthopaedic surgery. current practice and evolving applications. Bull Hosp Jt Dis (2013) 2015;73(4):257–68.

34. Lowe JT, Testa EJ, Li X, et al. Magnetic resonance imaging is comparable to computed tomography for determination of glenoid version but does not accurately distinguish between Walch B2 and C classifications. J Shoulder Elbow Surg 2017;26(4):669–73.

35. Scalise JJ, Codsi MJ, Bryan J, et al. The three-dimensional glenoid vault model can estimate normal glenoid version in osteoarthritis. J Shoulder Elbow Surg 2008;17(3):487–91.

36. Friedman RJ, Hawthorne KB, Genez BM. The use of computerized tomography in the measurement of glenoid version. J Bone Joint Surg Am 1992;74(7):1032–7.

37. Maurer A, Fucentese SF, Pfirrmann CW, et al. Assessment of glenoid inclination on routine clinical radiographs and computed tomography examinations of the shoulder. J Shoulder Elbow Surg 2012;21(8):1096–103.

38. Scalise JJ, Codsi MJ, Bryan J, et al. The influence of three-dimensional computed tomography images of the shoulder in preoperative planning for total shoulder arthroplasty. J Bone Joint Surg Am 2008; 90(11):2438–45.

39. Bryce CD, Davison AC, Lewis GS, et al. Two-dimensional glenoid version measurements vary with coronal and sagittal scapular rotation. J Bone Joint Surg Am 2010;92(3):692–9.

40. Kwon YW, Powell KA, Yum JK, et al. Use of three-dimensional computed tomography for the analysis of the glenoid anatomy. J Shoulder Elbow Surg 2005;14(1):85–90.

41. Bokor DJ, O'Sullivan MD, Hazan GJ. Variability of measurement of glenoid version on computed tomography scan. J Shoulder Elbow Surg 1999;8(6):595–8.

42. Denard PJ, Provencher MT, Lädermann A, et al. Version and inclination obtained with 3-dimensional planning in total shoulder arthroplasty: do different programs produce the same results? JSES Open Access 2018;2(4):200–4.

43. Erickson BJ, Chalmers PN, Denard P, et al. Does commercially available shoulder arthroplasty preoperative planning software agree with surgeon measurements of version, inclination, and subluxation? J Shoulder Elbow Surg 2021;30(2):413–20.

44. Nowak DD, Bahu MJ, Gardner TR, et al. Simulation of surgical glenoid resurfacing using three-dimensional computed tomography of the arthritic glenohumeral joint: the amount of glenoid retroversion that can be corrected. J Shoulder Elbow Surg 2009;18(5):680–8.

45. Clavert P, Millett PJ, Warner JJ. Glenoid resurfacing: what are the limits to asymmetric reaming for posterior erosion? J Shoulder Elbow Surg 2007; 16(6):843–8.

46. Sabesan V, Callanan M, Ho J, et al. Clinical and radiographic outcomes of total shoulder arthroplasty with bone graft for osteoarthritis with severe glenoid bone loss. J Bone Joint Surg Am 2013; 95(14):1290–6.

47. Knowles NK, Ferreira LM, Athwal GS. Augmented glenoid component designs for type B2 erosions:

a computational comparison by volume of bone removal and quality of remaining bone. J Shoulder Elbow Surg 2015;24(8):1218–26.

48. Rosenthal Y, Rettig SA, Virk MS, et al. Impact of preoperative 3-dimensional planning and intraoperative navigation of shoulder arthroplasty on implant selection and operative time: a single surgeon's experience. J Shoulder Elbow Surg 2020;29(12):2564–70.

49. Jacquot A, Gauci MO, Chaoui J, et al. Proper benefit of a three dimensional pre-operative planning software for glenoid component positioning in total shoulder arthroplasty. Int Orthop 2018;42(12):2897–906.

50. Throckmorton TW, Gulotta LV, Bonnarens FO, et al. Patient-specific targeting guides compared with traditional instrumentation for glenoid component placement in shoulder arthroplasty: a multisurgeon study in 70 arthritic cadaver specimens. J Shoulder Elbow Surg 2015;24(6):965–71.

51. Berhouet J, Gulotta LV, Dines DM, et al. Preoperative planning for accurate glenoid component positioning in reverse shoulder arthroplasty. Orthop Traumatol Surg Res 2017;103(3):407–13.

52. Berhouet J, Jacquot A, Walch G, et al. Preoperative planning of baseplate position in reverse shoulder arthroplasty: still no consensus on lateralization, version and inclination. Orthop Traumatol Surg Res 2022;108(3):103115.

53. Lee CS, Davis SM, Lane CJ, et al. Reliability and accuracy of digital templating for the humeral component of total shoulder arthroplasty. Shoulder Elbow 2015;7(1):29–35.

54. Freehill MT, Weick JW, Ponce BA, et al. Anatomic total shoulder arthroplasty: component size prediction with 3-dimensional pre-operative digital planning. J Shoulder Elb Arthroplast 2022;6. 24715492221098818.

55. Poltaretskyi S, Chaoui J, Mayya M, et al. Prediction of the pre-morbid 3D anatomy of the proximal humerus based on statistical shape modelling. Bone Joint J 2017;99-B(7):927–33.

56. Giannotti S, Sacchetti F, Citarelli C, et al. Single-use, patient-specific instrumentation technology in knee arthroplasty: a comparative study between standard instrumentation and PSI efficiency system. Musculoskelet Surg 2020;104(2):195–200.

57. Gomes NS. Patient-specific instrumentation for total shoulder arthroplasty. EFORT Open Rev 2017;1(5):177–82.

58. Yam MGJ, Chao JYY, Leong C, et al. 3D printed patient specific customised surgical jig for reverse shoulder arthroplasty, a cost effective and accurate solution. J Clin Orthop Trauma 2021;21:101503.

59. Hendel MD, Bryan JA, Barsoum WK, et al. Comparison of patient-specific instruments with standard surgical instruments in determining glenoid component position: a randomized prospective clinical trial. J Bone Joint Surg Am 2012;94(23):2167–75.

60. Iannotti JP, Weiner S, Rodriguez E, et al. Three-dimensional imaging and templating improve glenoid implant positioning. J Bone Joint Surg Am 2015;97(8):651–8.

61. Cabarcas BC, Cvetanovich GL, Gowd AK, et al. Accuracy of patient-specific instrumentation in shoulder arthroplasty: a systematic review and meta-analysis. JSES Open Access 2019;3(3):117–29.

62. Villatte G, Muller AS, Pereira B, et al. Use of patient-specific instrumentation (PSI) for glenoid component positioning in shoulder arthroplasty. A systematic review and meta-analysis. PLoS One 2018;13(8):e0201759.

63. Darwood A, Hurst SA, Villatte G, et al. Novel robotic technology for the rapid intraoperative manufacture of patient-specific instrumentation allowing for improved glenoid component accuracy in shoulder arthroplasty: a cadaveric study. J Shoulder Elbow Surg 2022;31(3):561–70.

64. Walch G, Vezeridis PS, Boileau P, et al. Three-dimensional planning and use of patient-specific guides improve glenoid component position: an in vitro study. J Shoulder Elbow Surg 2015;24(2):302–9.

65. Moineau G, Levigne C, Boileau P, et al, French Society for Shoulder & Elbow (SOFEC). Three-dimensional measurement method of arthritic glenoid cavity morphology: feasibility and reproducibility. Orthop Traumatol Surg Res 2012;98(6 Suppl):S139–45.

66. Gregory TM, Sankey A, Augereau B, et al. Accuracy of glenoid component placement in total shoulder arthroplasty and its effect on clinical and radiological outcome in a retrospective, longitudinal, monocentric open study. PLoS One 2013;8(10):e75791.

67. Davis ET, Gallie P, Macgroarty K, et al. The accuracy of image-free computer navigation in the placement of the femoral component of the Birmingham Hip Resurfacing: a cadaver study. J Bone Joint Surg Br 2007;89(4):557–60.

68. Lützner J, Krummenauer F, Wolf C, et al. Computer-assisted and conventional total knee replacement: a comparative, prospective, randomised study with radiological and CT evaluation. J Bone Joint Surg Br 2008;90(8):1039–44.

69. Stindel E, Merloz P, Graf P, et al. 'expérience de la navigation chirurgicale dans l'ouest [computer assisted orthopedics surgery]. Rev Chir Orthop Reparatrice Appar Mot 2007;93(4 Suppl):2S11–32.

70. Victor J, Hoste D. Image-based computer-assisted total knee arthroplasty leads to lower variability in coronal alignment. Clin Orthop Relat Res 2004;428:131–9.

71. Lung TS, Cruickshank D, Grant HJ, et al. Factors contributing to glenoid baseplate micromotion in reverse shoulder arthroplasty: a biomechanical study. J Shoulder Elbow Surg 2019;28(4):648–53.

72. Jahic D, Suero EM, Marjanovic B. The use of computer navigation and patient specific instrumentation in shoulder arthroplasty: everyday practice, just for special cases or actually teaching a surgeon? Acta Inform Med 2021;29(2):130–3.

73. Verborgt O, Vanhees M, Heylen S, et al. Computer navigation and patient-specific instrumentation in shoulder arthroplasty. Sports Med Arthrosc Rev 2014;22(4):e42–9.

74. Edwards TB, Gartsman GM, O'Connor DP, et al. Safety and utility of computer-aided shoulder arthroplasty. J Shoulder Elbow Surg 2008;17(3):503–8.

75. Nguyen D, Ferreira LM, Brownhill JR, et al. Improved accuracy of computer assisted glenoid implantation in total shoulder arthroplasty: an in-vitro randomized controlled trial. J Shoulder Elbow Surg 2009;18(6):907–14.

76. Aminov O, Regan W, Giles JW, et al. Targeting repeatability of a less obtrusive surgical navigation procedure for total shoulder arthroplasty. Int J Comput Assist Radiol Surg 2022;17(2):283–93.

77. Colasanti GB, Moreschini F, Cataldi C, et al. GPS guided reverse shoulder arthroplasty. Acta Biomed 2020;91(4-S):204–8.

78. Verborgt O, De Smedt T, Vanhees M, et al. Accuracy of placement of the glenoid component in reversed shoulder arthroplasty with and without navigation. J Shoulder Elbow Surg 2011;20(1):21–6.

79. Kircher J, Wiedemann M, Magosch P, et al. Improved accuracy of glenoid positioning in total shoulder arthroplasty with intraoperative navigation: a prospective-randomized clinical study. J Shoulder Elbow Surg 2009;18(4):515–20.

80. Wang AW, Hayes A, Gibbons R, et al. Computer navigation of the glenoid component in reverse total shoulder arthroplasty: a clinical trial to evaluate the learning curve. J Shoulder Elbow Surg 2020;29(3):617–23.

81. Schoch BS, Haupt E, Leonor T, et al. Computer navigation leads to more accurate glenoid targeting during total shoulder arthroplasty compared with 3-dimensional preoperative planning alone. J Shoulder Elbow Surg 2020;29(11):2257–63.

82. Sadoghi P, Vavken J, Leithner A, et al. Benefit of intraoperative navigation on glenoid component positioning during total shoulder arthroplasty. Arch Orthop Trauma Surg 2015;135(1):41–7.

83. Burns DM, Frank T, Whyne CM, et al. Glenoid component positioning and guidance techniques in anatomic and reverse total shoulder arthroplasty: A systematic review and meta-analysis. Shoulder Elbow 2019;11(2 Suppl):16–28.

84. Moreschini F, Colasanti GB, Cataldi C, et al. Pre-operative CT-based planning integrated with intra-operative navigation in reverse shoulder arthroplasty: data acquisition and analysis protocol, and preliminary results of navigated versus conventional surgery. Dose Response 2020;18(4).1559325820970832.

85. Hones KM, King JJ, Schoch BS, et al. The in vivo impact of computer navigation on screw number and length in reverse total shoulder arthroplasty. J Shoulder Elbow Surg 2021;30(10):e629–35.

86. Sprowls GR, Wilson CD, Stewart W, et al. Intraoperative navigation and preoperative templating software are associated with increased glenoid baseplate screw length and use of augmented baseplates in reverse total shoulder arthroplasty. JSES Int 2020;5(1):102–8.

87. Suter T, Kolz CW, Tashjian RZ, et al. Humeral head osteotomy in shoulder arthroplasty: a comparison between anterosuperior and inferoanterior resection techniques. J Shoulder Elbow Surg 2017;26(2):343–51.

88. Geervliet PC, Willems JH, Sierevelt IN, et al. Over-stuffing in resurfacing hemiarthroplasty is a potential risk for failure. J Orthop Surg Res 2019;14(1):474.

89. Cavanagh J, Lockhart J, Langohr GDG, et al. A comparison of patient-specific instrumentation to navigation for conducting humeral head osteotomies during shoulder arthroplasty. JSES Int 2021;5(5):875–80.

90. Jud L, Fotouhi J, Andronic O, et al. Applicability of augmented reality in orthopedic surgery - a systematic review. BMC Musculoskelet Disord 2020;21(1):103.

91. Berhouet J, Slimane M, Facomprez M, et al. Views on a new surgical assistance method for implanting the glenoid component during total shoulder arthroplasty. Part 2: From three-dimensional reconstruction to augmented reality: feasibility study. Orthop Traumatol Surg Res 2019;105(2):211–8.

92. Kriechling P, Loucas R, Loucas M, et al. Augmented reality through head-mounted display for navigation of baseplate component placement in reverse total shoulder arthroplasty: a cadaveric study. Arch Orthop Trauma Surg 2021. https://doi.org/10.1007/s00402-021-04025-5. published online ahead of print, 2021 Jul 2.

93. Kriechling P, Roner S, Liebmann F, et al. Augmented reality for base plate component placement in reverse total shoulder arthroplasty: a feasibility study. Arch Orthop Trauma Surg 2021;141(9):1447–53.

94. Schlueter-Brust K, Henckel J, Katinakis F, et al. Augmented-reality-assisted K-wire placement for

glenoid component positioning in reversed shoulder arthroplasty: a proof-of-concept study. J Pers Med 2021;11(8):777.

95. Gregory TM, Gregory J, Sledge J, et al. Surgery guided by mixed reality: presentation of a proof of concept. Acta Orthop 2018;89(5):480–3.

96. Rojas JT, Lädermann A, Ho SWL, et al. Glenoid component placement assisted by augmented reality through a head-mounted display during reverse shoulder arthroplasty. Arthrosc Tech 2022; 11(5):e863–74.

97. Ponce et al teaching in SA, Ponce BA, Menendez ME, et al. Emerging technology in surgical education: combining real-time augmented reality and wearable computing devices. Orthopedics 2014;37:751–7.

Foot and Ankle

Advances in Cartilage Repair

Mohammad T. Azam, BS[a], James J. Butler, MB BCh[a], Matthew L. Duenes, MD[a], Thomas W. McAllister, MBBS[a,b], Raymond C. Walls[a], Arianna L. Gianakos, DO[a], John G. Kennedy, MD, MCh, MMSc, FFSEM, FRCS (Orth)[a,*]

KEYWORDS

- Ankle osteochondral lesion • Microfracture • Autologous osteochondral transplantation
- Biologics

KEY POINTS

- Osteochondral lesions of the ankle joint are difficult to manage because of the poor regenerative ability of the articular cartilage and, thus, are typically managed surgically.
- Lesions that are small (<100 mm^2 or <10 mm) can be treated with less invasive procedures such as arthroscopic debridement, anterograde drilling, scaffold-based therapies, and augmentation with biological adjuvants.
- Caution should be taken when utilizing bone marrow stimulation via microfracture as it produces an unstable fibrocartilage infill and damages the underlying subchondral plate.
- For patients with large lesions (>100 mm^2 or >10 mm), cystic lesions, uncontained lesions, or patients in whom prior bone marrow stimulation has failed, management with autologous osteochondral transplantation is indicated.
- Biological adjuvants such as platelet-rich plasma, concentrated bone marrow aspirate, and hyaluronic acid can accelerate the regenerative process, but definitive guidelines regarding their role are yet to be determined.

 Video content accompanies this article at http://www.orthopedic.theclinics.com.

INTRODUCTION

Osteochondral lesions (OCLs) of the ankle joint are characterized by injury to the articular cartilage and/or underlying subchondral bone.[1] This debilitating pathology is often preceded by acute trauma such as ankle sprains or fractures, or can be precipitated by chronic, repetitive microtrauma to the joint.[1] Nontraumatic etiologies include spontaneous necrosis, generalized ligamentous laxity, systemic vasculopathies, metabolic disorders, and embolic disease.[2] Patients present with deep ankle pain, swelling, altered gait, and concomitant ankle instability.[1]

Diagnosis is often delayed because of a low index of suspicion together with poor sensitivity of plain film radiographs for detecting OCLs.[3] Although computed tomography (CT) scans allow for excellent visualization of the subchondral bone, they are limited in their evaluation of the articular cartilage.[4] MRI is the gold standard imaging modality and has a sensitivity and specificity of 96% for detecting OCLs at the ankle.[4] It permits detailed assessment of the articular cartilage (Table 1), the subchondral bone, and any concomitant soft tissue pathology. However, MRI may overestimate the size of the lesion because of subchondral bone

[a] Foot and Ankle Division, Department of Orthopaedic Surgery, NYU Langone Health, 171 Delancey Street, New York, NY 10002, USA; [b] University of Cambrdige School of Clinical Medicine, Box 111 Cambridge Biomedical Campus, Cambridge CB2 0SP, UK
* Corresponding author.
E-mail address: john.kennedy@nyulangone.org

Orthop Clin N Am 54 (2023) 227–236
https://doi.org/10.1016/j.ocl.2022.11.007
0030-5898/23/© 2022 Elsevier Inc. All rights reserved.

Table 1
MRI classification for osteochondral lesions of the talus

Stage	Definition
1	Articular cartilage damage only
2a	Cartilage injury with underlying fracture and surrounding bony edema
2b	Stage 2a without surrounding bony edema
3	Detached but nondisplaced fragment
4	Detached and displaced fragment
5	Subchondral cyst formation

marrow edema that extends beyond the margin of the lesion.[4]

Outcomes following conservative management of ankle OCLs are unsatisfactory because of the poor regenerative biology of the avascular articular cartilage and limited blood supply to the talus and subchondral bone.[5,6] Conventionally, surgical management of ankle OCLs is determined by lesion size.[6] Surgical options described for smaller lesions (<10 mm in diameter or <100 mm^2) include arthroscopic debridement, bone marrow stimulation (BMS), scaffold-based therapies and augmentation with biological adjuvants such as platelet-rich plasma (PRP), concentrated bone marrow aspirate (CBMA), or hyaluronic acid (HA).[6,7] Replacement procedures, such as autologous osteochondral transplantation (AOT), are indicated for patients with large lesions (>10 mm in diameter or >100 mm^2), cystic lesions, uncontained lesions, or for patients who have failed a prior reparative procedure such as BMS.[8]

This article describes the most recent clinical evidence regarding the various treatment modalities for ankle OCLs. It also details the limitations associated with each therapeutic option.

REPARATIVE

BMS via microfracture is a widely used surgical intervention for OCLs of the ankle and knee joint.[9] Various surgical instruments such as a pick, awl, or drill are used to perforate the subchondral plate stimulating the aggregation of mesenchymal stem cells (MSCs) at the defect site, and, in response to growth factors, BMS promotes the generation of fibrocartilaginous tissue.[10,11] BMS has been used in lesions of varying sizes; however, the International Congress on Cartilage Repair of the Ankle consensus

meeting in 2018 demonstrated that BMS may not be suitable in patients with an OCL greater than 100 mm^2 or greater than 10 mm in diameter.[12] Although favorable results have been demonstrated following BMS for smaller lesions at short- to midterm follow-up,[13] there remains concern regarding degradation of the repair tissue over time.

The hyaline cartilage at the ankle joint is predominantly composed of type-II collagen and high levels of proteoglycans.[14] The fibrocartilage tissue produced by BMS is histologically comparable to native hyaline cartilage during the initial 6 weeks following BMS.[15] Eventually, numerous biological alterations occur, including de-differentiation of type-II collagen into type-I collagen, reduced expression of proteoglycans, and tissue fibrillation, ultimately producing a hyaline-like substance.[15] This hyaline-like material is less resilient, less durable and, ultimately, inferior in comparison to the native hyaline cartilage and is susceptible to degradation from shear forces.[10] Although improvement in subjective outcomes have been reported, numerous studies found degradation of the reparative fibrous cartilage over time. Lee and colleagues[16] performed second-look arthroscopies 1 year following BMS and found that 30% of their cohort demonstrated adequate integration of the repair tissue with the adjacent native tissue. Furthermore, MRI obtained 5 years following BMS demonstrated fibrillation of the fibrocartilage tissue in all patients.[17]

The subchondral plate and subchondral bone play a crucial role in the preservation of the ankle joint. The subchondral bone functions as a structural scaffold bearing 30% of the compressive load through the joint, compared to the 1% to 3% of load absorbed by the articular cartilage.[5] In addition, the subchondral bone communicates with the articular cartilage via cross-talk to facilitate a variety of signaling pathways.[18] Concerns have been raised regarding the integrity of the subchondral plate following BMS. Chen and colleagues[19] conducted a rabbit study and found that microfracture induced bone fracturing and compaction with profound osteocyte necrosis in the adjacent bone. Orth and colleagues[20] performed BMS in sheep and reported a reduction in bone volume and trabecular thickness, with an increase in subchondral cysts and intralesional osteophytes. In addition, a systematic review by Seow and colleagues[21] found that BMS produced significant histological changes and reduced density of the architecture of the deep subchondral bone. These findings have been replicated in clinical studies. Kennedy and colleagues followed a cohort of 42 patients who underwent BMS for OCLs of the talus (OLTs). Despite an initial improvement in foot and ankle outcome score (FAOS), there was a reduction in FAOS at final follow-up of 51.7 months.[5] Furthermore, there was a significant decrease in the subchondral bone health score as assessed via MRI at final follow-up with increased subchondral cyst formation.[5]

Unfortunately, the methodological quality of many of the studies is poor, with marked heterogeneity and under-reporting of data between the studies. Therefore, caution must be taken when evaluating these outcomes.

REGENERATIVE

Regenerative techniques for ankle OCLs include autologous chondrocyte implantation (ACI), matrix-induced autologous chondrocyte implantation (MACI), and autologous matrix-induced chondrogenesis (AMIC). These procedures are often utilized after failed microfracture or for larger lesions not amenable to BMS.

ACI is a 2-stage procedure that was first used to manage chondral defects in the knee.[22] The first stage of ACI involves harvesting hyaline cartilage from a non-weight bearing portion of the knee or the anterior talus. The harvested chondrocytes are then isolated, and the extracellular matrix is enzymatically removed. The cells are then cultured and expanded in vitro for 11 to 21 days, where the cells dedifferentiate and return to a fetal stage. During the second stage, the cells are directly implanted into the OCL, and a periosteal patch is sewn over the defect to contain the suspended cells and provide growth factors to promote chondrogenesis. Brittberg and colleagues[22] performed ACI in patients with full-thickness knee OCLs. The authors reported good subjective outcomes at final follow-up with approximately 80% of knees expressing type-II collagen with the appearance of hyaline cartilage. Overall clinical success at 10-year follow-up has been reported 89.9%; however, the procedure has multiple drawbacks.[23,24] ACI requires 2 procedures and a wide exposure to perform the periosteal sleeve, which includes osteotomy and graft site morbidity. Additionally, in a study by Kwak and colleagues,[23] 86% of patients required removal of hardware, and 38% had periosteal softening and hypertrophy.

MACI is a regenerative technique that embeds cultured autogenous chondrocytes in a matrix of either type-I/III collagen, hyaluronan, or polyglycolic acid, which is secured with fibrin glue.[25] Implantation can be performed arthroscopically, avoiding periosteal harvest morbidity and reliance on suture fixation. There are more viable cells delivered to the lesion compared with ACI, which is susceptible to leakage and uneven distribution. Patients undergoing MACI have comparable clinical scores to ACI.[26] Most patients have mean improvements in AOFAS scores ranging from 13 to 24 up to 12-year follow-up.[25,26] Similar to ACI, MRI findings do not necessarily correlate with the clinical outcomes. Although clinical results of MACI procedures are overall positive, limitations remain, most notably the need for 2 procedures and cost.

AMIC is a single-stage cartilage repair technique with promising results.[27] The procedure involves microfracture with application of an exogenous scaffold, such as a collagen type-I/III bilayer. By utilizing a matrix, the chondrogenic clot induced by BMS is covered, stabilized, and provides an early 3-dimensional scaffold to seed MSCs. Additionally, biological augments can be included in the scaffold via CBMA or PRP to further promote hyaline cartilage formation. In a case series performed by Weigelt and colleagues,[28] 33 patients underwent an open AMIC procedure with a mean follow-up of 4.7 years, mean AOFAS score of 93, and a 79% return to sport rate. The matrix can be loaded into lesions arthroscopically, with reported AOFAS scores of 20 point improvements at 2 years.[29] When directly comparing ACI, MACI, and AMIC for OLTs, all 3 groups have similar clinical outcome scores at short-term follow-up.[30] Additionally, second-look arthroscopy has demonstrated continuous, intact cartilaginous layers filling the defects with type-II collagen identified in biopsies. AMIC appears to be an attractive alternative to ACI and MACI, because it is a single procedure, more cost-effective, and circumvents morbidity associated with grafts and harvesting chondrocytes. However, longer term follow-up is still limited.

Extracellular matrix allografts (ECMA) can also be utilized to augment BMS. BioCartilage (Arthrex Inc., Nas, Florida) is a dehydrated, micronized allogenic cartilage ECMA that contains type-II collagen and proteoglycans.[31] It provides a scaffold for MSCs to infiltrate and produce a higher quality cartilage infill. Fortier and colleagues[32] reported in an equine model microfracture augmented with PRP, and BioCartilage produced an infill with significantly better ICRA histology score and MRI T2 relaxation times than microfracture alone. Furthermore, Kennedy and colleagues[33] utilized

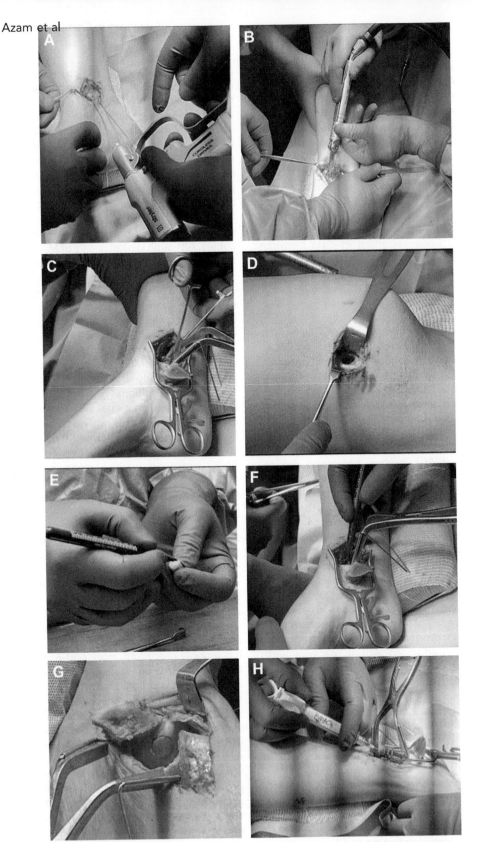

Fig. 1. (*A*) Prior to making the osteotomy cut, a provisional K wire is drilled into the medial malleolus at angle of 30° relative to the long axis of the tibia. Next, the medial malleolus is predrilled with 2 parallel fixation holes (*B*) An oscillating saw is used to create a Chevron-type osteotomy, which is continued for 7/8s of the bone. The saw is stopped at the level of the subchondral bone. The osteotomy is then completed using a sharp half-inch osteotome.

BioCartilage and CBMA to augment BMS. At 20 months follow-up on MRI, they found 87.6% of patients who had BioCartilage had comte infill of their defect compared with 46.5% for BMS without BioCartilage. Longer-term studies will be needed to determine whether ECMA provides robust cartilage repair that will be sustained over a longer period than BMS alone.

REPLACEMENT

Replacement strategies including AOT are indicated in patients with larger lesions (area >100 mm^2 or diameter >10 mm), cystic lesions, uncontained lesions, or patients who have failed previous BMS.[8] AOT offers many advantages to reparative and regenerative techniques by removing and replacing not only the damaged overlying cartilage, but also the critical subchondral plate and bone, providing a more comprehensive solution.[2] Autograft transplant is the senior surgeon's preferred method in comparison to allograft transfer. In their comparative study, Kennedy and colleagues reported poorer clinical outcomes and poor host graft integration on MRI in the allograft group.[34] Similarly, a meta-analysis by Migliorini and colleagues[35] found autograft to have lower failure and rates compared with allograft at midterm follow-up.

AOT involves resection of the diseased cartilage and underlying subchondral bone in a cylinder shape from the talus and is subsequently replaced with an autograft harvested from the non-weight bearing portion of the lateral femoral condyle. OLTs that are medially located can be accessed through a chevron-type medial malleolar osteotomy. For lateral lesions, a tibial trapezoidal osteotomy can be utilized to gain access to all but the most posterior lesions, avoiding a fibular takedown (Fig. 1).[36]

Several studies have reported favorable outcomes following AOT (Fig. 2). In a cohort of 72 patients, Murawski and colleagues[36] reported a significant improved in FAOS scores at

28 months follow-up and an average RTS of 12 weeks. Furthermore, T2 mapping on MRI 1 year after AOT demonstrated restoration of the radius of curvature and color stratification similar to that of native cartilage. Similarly, for larger OLTs in the athletic population, Nguyen and colleagues[37] reported significant improvement in visual analog scale (VAS) scores at 45 months follow-up, with 87% of patients returning to previous level of sport.

BIOLOGICAL ADJUVANTS
Platelet-Rich Plasma

Platelet-rich plasma (PRP) is an autologous blood product generated by centrifugation of peripheral blood to produce an increased concentration of platelets. PRP consists of growth factors including fibroblast growth factor, vascular endothelial growth factor, insulin-like growth factor, platelet-derived growth factor, and transforming growth factor-β (TGF-β1).[38] These growth factors and cytokines play key roles in MSC chemotaxis, target cell activation, cell proliferation, neoangiogenesis, and cartilage matrix production, and provide an additional immuno-modulatory benefit.[38]

Several studies have examined the potential chondroprotective effects of PRP when used in conjunction with either BMS or AOT. The combination of BMS and PRP has been shown to promote a supportive biological environment encouraging chondrocyte synthesis and an increase in type-II collagen deposition.[39] A randomized controlled trial (RCT) by Gormeli and colleagues[40] showed a statistically significant increase in AOFAS scores and decreased VAS scores for patients with OLTs treated with BMS and PRP compared to BMS and HA injections and a saline control group. Furthermore, an RCT by Guney and colleagues[41] found significantly improved clinical outcomes in the cohort treated with BMS and PRP compared with BMS alone. However, a systematic review by Seow and colleagues[42] found there were a limited

---

(C) Following release and reflection of the bone and soft tissue, a modified retractor is used to facilitate adequate exposure of the medial aspect of the talar surface. For lateral lesions, a tibial trapezoidal osteotomy can be utilized to gain access to all but the most posterior lesions, avoiding a fibular takedown. (D) A mini-open arthrotomy is used to harvest the donor plug from the lateral non-weight bearing portion of the ipsilateral femoral condyle, which is then bathed in CBMA. For lesions greater than 10 mm in diameter, 2 grafts are used. The 2 grafts are placed side by side in a figure-of-8 or half-moon configuration, which allows the fibrocartilage to fill in the nonadjacent space of the graft. The base of the graft recipient is overdrilled by 2 mm using an acorn-shaped drill tip so as to maintain articular congruency during the postoperative maturation and remodeling process. (E–G) Both the donor plug and the highest point of the peripheral margin of the OCL are marked with a pen. The graft should be gently placed into the most congruent position possible. (H) The ankle is then injected with CBMA.

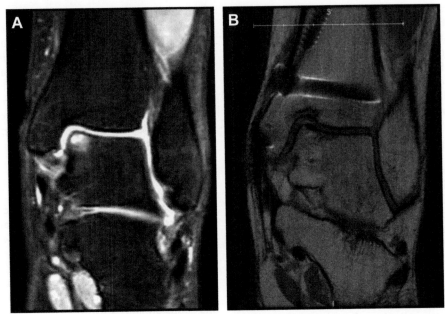

Fig. 2. (A) 21-year-old female runner presented with a 1-year history of left ankle pain following an acute ankle inversion injury. Her MRI (A) demonstrated a 12 mm × 6 mm cystic osteochondral lesion at the shoulder of the medial talus. She subsequently underwent autologous osteochondral transplantation with injection of CBMA. She had a repeat MRI (B) of the left ankle at 4 months postoperatively, which demonstrated satisfactory integration of the donor graft into the recipient talar dome.

number of comparative studies evaluating the role of PRP in BMS, warranting future research. There appears to be limited data regarding the role of PRP as an adjunct to AOT procedures. Boakye and colleagues[43] found elevated levels of TGF-β1 in rabbits that underwent AOT procedure with concomitant PRP compared with those that did not receive PRP. Additionally, Smyth and colleagues[44] showed improved graft integration and higher mean ICRS scores in those who underwent AOT with adjuvant PRP compared with AOT alone.

In summary, PRP is a readily available resource that promotes cartilage repair and type-II collagen deposition supported by basic scientific princis and clinical research. However, there is significant variability between patients, preparation techniques, and overall poor quality of evidence, which makes analysis of the overall literature challenging.[45]

Concentrated Bone Marrow Aspirate

Traditional theory suggested that MSCs differentiated directly into osteoblasts and chondrocytes to support cartilage repair.[46] However, new evidence proposes that most MSCs are engulfed by macrophages and form a secretome–a paracrine signaling apparatus–which promotes regenerative processes via immunomodulatory effects such as down regulation of proinflammatory interleukin (IL)-1β gene expression.[47] CBMA contains a potent anti-inflammatory, IL-1 receptor antagonist protein, which prevents activation of inflammatory cytokine cascades.[47] CBMA contains many growth factors such as TGFβ, which promotes chondrogenic differentiation of MSCs and type-II collagen formation.[48]

CBMA is a useful adjunct to BMS, as the addition of MSCs and growth factors into a cartilage defect promotes a hyaline-like repair and increased type-II collagen deposition. This has been demonstrated in animal models, particularly in equine medicine.[49,50] Fortier and colleagues[49] compared the results of microfracture alone to microfracture and CBMA in an equine model and found improved radiological and histological repair in the CBMA group. The use of CBMA in conjunction with BMS has produced encouraging outcomes.[14,51] Hannon and colleagues[14] compared outcomes for patients with OLTs treated with BMS and CMBA or BMS alone and found significantly improved FAOS and MOCART (magnetic resonance observation of cartilage repair tissue) scores in the CBMA group. Radiologically the

CBMA group showed increased infilling of the lesion, and over 95% had comte integration, with lower rates of fissuring than the BMS-only group. Murphy and colleagues[51] found a statistically significant decrease in the revision rate for the BMS and CBMA cohort.

Mercer and colleagues[52] found that in patients treated with AOT for OLTs, the addition of CBMA alone produced comparable results to CBMA plus ECMA, suggesting that CBMA alone provides sufficient augmentation for successful graft integration. Furthermore, Kennedy and colleagues[53] demonstrated that CBMA reduces postoperative subchondral cysts following AOT.

Hyaluronic Acid

HA is a high-molecular weight polysaccharide glycosaminoglycan. HA is found naturally in the synovial fluid and is responsible for maintaining the viscoelastic properties of joints, reducing friction, and transmitting shear forces.[7]

In addition to its beneficial rheological properties, HA plays an important biological role enhancing proliferation of chondrocytes and stimulating chondroitin sulfate synthesis, an important component of proteoglycans.[7] HA has been proposed as a useful adjunct to BMS for cartilage repair[54] and has exhibited chondroprotective and anti-inflammatory properties in animal studies.[55] This is supported by clinical outcome data, which report improved functional and MRI outcomes for patients undergoing BMS, although HA appears to be inferior to PRP in this regard.[40]

Recent advances include the use of HA-based cell-free bioscaffolds (HACS) such as Hyalofast (Anika Therapeutics Inc., Bedford, Massachusetts), which trap MSCs.[56] This supports a paracrine signaling environment that mediates angiogenesis, cell survival, and differentiation, improving the healing capacity of the cartilage and preventing fibrosis.[57] Histological studies show an increase in hyaline-like cartilage formation.[57] Clinical data report improvements in pain scores and radiological outcomes, especially when HACS is used in conjunction with BMS and CBMA.[58]

FUTURE DEVELOPMENTS

In-office nano-arthroscopy (IONA) is a novel needle arthroscopic system that facilitates inspection, evaluation, and treatment of a diseased joint using a 2.2 mm arthroscope and sheath.[59] These procedures are conducted with wide awake local anesthetic no tourniquet (WALANT),

facilitating rapid recovery and return to daily activities. The IONA system utilizes an optic chip at the tip of the camera, which provides high-quality, high-resolution (400 × 400 pixel) images with a 120° field of view.[59] In addition, surgical tools such as graspers, shavers, burrs, probes, scissors, and resectors can be used with the IONA technology to manage the specific pathology. IONA procedures are carried out at the bedside with the patient fully conscious, providing feedback to the surgeon.

The exact role of IONA for the management of OCLs of the ankle joint has not yet been determined, primarily because of its recent resurgence. IONA can directly visualize the OCL and may offer a more precise assessment of the size of the lesion than that obtained on conventional MRI. In addition, IONA can be used to inspect the entire ankle joint to identify and treat any concomitant pathologies that may not have been captured on MRI. At their institution, the authors have utilized IONA to directly treat smaller OCLs with debridement, drilling, and delivery of biological adjuvants such as PRP, CBMA, and scaffold-based therapies such as ECMA (Video 1).

Ankle impingement secondary to excessive scar tissue formation is commonly encountered following routine ankle surgery, including surgical intervention for OCLs of the ankle joint.[59] Patients frequently present with ankle pain with restricted dorsiflexion at the ankle joint. A recent study by Colasanti and colleagues[59] described the utility of IONA in the debridement of this cicatrized tissue. This retrospective study of 31 patients reported significant improvement in PROMIS (Patient-Reported Outcomes Measurement Information System) scores and FAOS scores at final follow-up, with 96% returning to sport at a mean time of 3.9 weeks. In patients who present with ankle impingement following surgical intervention for ankle OCLs, IONA can be an effective tool to simultaneously resect the excessive scar tissue and to evaluate the integrity of the repaired articular cartilage and/or autograft (Video 2).

SUMMARY

An osteochondral lesion of the ankle joint is a challenging pathology to treat in light of the limited self-regenerative capacity of the articular cartilage. Smaller lesions (<100 mm^2 or <10 mm) can be managed with less invasive procedures such as arthroscopic debridement, anterograde drilling, and augmentation with biological adjuvants. Care should be taken when considering treating the OCL with BMS because of the inferior fibrocartilage infill that is produced together with the damage to the underlying subchondral plate. Large lesions (>100 mm^2 or >10 mm), cystic lesions, uncontained lesions, or a failed prior BMS procedure warrant a replacement procedure such as an AOT. AOT has been shown to produce excellent results at long-term follow-up, with reported success rates of over 90%. Biological adjuvants such as PRP, CBMA, and HA are promising treatment modalities that can augment the cartilaginous regenerative process, but the precise indication for each biologic is yet to be determined.

CLINICS CARE POINTS

- The current gold standard diagnostic imaging modality is MRI, but it can overestimate the size of the OCL.

- Lesion size is a major factor in deciding the appropriate treatment strategy

- Smaller lesions (<100 mm^2 or <10 mm) can be managed with less invasive procedures such as arthroscopic debridement, anterograde drilling, and augmentation with biological adjuvants.

- BMS via microfracture damages the underlying subchondral plate and also produces an inferior fibrocartilage infill that degenerates over time.

- Indications for AOT include: large lesions (>100 mm^2 or >10 mm), cystic lesions, uncontained lesions, or patients who have failed prior BMS.

- Biological adjuvants such as PRP, CBMA, and HA have been demonstrated to accelerate the regenerative process, but definitive guidelines regarding their role have yet to be determined.

DISCLOSURE

The authors report the following potential conflicts of interest or sources of funding: J.G. Kennedy is a consultant to Arteriocyte Industries (Isto Biologics) and Arthrex Inc., and receives support from Ohnell Family Foundation and Mr. and Mrs. Michael J. Levitt. J.G. Kennedy reports as a board or committee member for the American Orthopaedic Foot and Ankle Society, European Society of Sports Traumatology, Knee Surgery and Arthroscopy, Ankle and Foot Associates, and International Society for Cartilage Repair of the Ankle.

SUPPLEMENTARY DATA

Supmentary data related to this article can be found online at https://doi.org/10.1016/j.ocl. 2022.11.007.

REFERENCES

1. Barbier O, Amouyel T, de l'Escalopier N, et al. Osteochondral lesion of the talus: what are we talking about? Orthop Traumatol Surg Res 2021; 107(8s):103068.

2. O'Loughlin PF, Heyworth BE, Kennedy JG. Current concepts in the diagnosis and treatment of osteochondral lesions of the ankle. Am J Sports Med 2010;38(2):392–404.

3. Hamilton C, Burgul R, Kourkounis G, et al. Osteochondral defects of the talus: radiological appearance and surgical candidate profiling - A retrospective analysis. Foot (Edinb) 2021;46:101767.

4. Looze CA, Capo J, Ryan MK, et al. Evaluation and management of osteochondral lesions of the talus. Cartilage 2017;8(1):19–30.

5. Shimozono Y, Coale M, Yasui Y, et al. Subchondral bone degradation after microfracture for osteochondral lesions of the talus: an MRI analysis. Am J Sports Med 2018;46(3):642–8.

6. Lan T, McCarthy HS, Hulme CH, et al. The management of talar osteochondral lesions - current concepts. J Arthrosc Jt Surg 2021;8(3):231–7.

7. Kawasaki K, Ochi M, Uchio Y, et al. Hyaluronic acid enhances proliferation and chondroitin sulfate synthesis in cultured chondrocytes embedded in collagen gels. J Cell Physiol 1999;179(2):142–8.

8. Ramponi L, Yasui Y, Murawski CD, et al. Lesion size is a predictor of clinical outcomes after bone marrow stimulation for osteochondral lesions of the talus: a systematic review. Am J Sports Med 2017;45(7):1698–705.

9. Park JH, Park KH, Cho JY, et al. Bone marrow stimulation for osteochondral lesions of the talus: are clinical outcomes maintained 10 years later? Am J Sports Med 2021;49(5):1220–6.

10. Murawski CD, Foo LF, Kennedy JG. A review of arthroscopic bone marrow stimulation techniques of the talus: the good, the bad, and the causes for concern. Cartilage 2010;1(2):137–44.

11. Steadman JR, Rodkey WG, Rodrigo JJ. Microfracture: surgical technique and rehabilitation to treat chondral defects. Clin Orthop Relat Res 2001;(391 Suppl):S362–9. https://doi.org/10.1097/00003086-200110001-00033.

12. Smyth NA, Murawski CD, Adams SB Jr, et al. Osteochondral allograft: proceedings of the international consensus meeting on cartilage repair of the ankle. Foot Ankle Int 2018;39(1_Suppl):35s–40s.

13. Rikken QGH, Dahmen J, Reilingh ML, et al. Outcomes of bone marrow stimulation for secondary osteochondral lesions of the talus equal outcomes for primary lesions. Cartilage 2021;13(1_Suppl): 1429s–37s.

14. Hannon CP, Ross KA, Murawski CD, et al. Arthroscopic bone marrow stimulation and concentrated bone marrow aspirate for osteochondral lesions of the talus: a case-control study of functional and magnetic resonance observation of cartilage repair tissue outcomes. Arthroscopy 2016;32(2):339–47.

15. Shapiro F, Koide S, Glimcher MJ. Cell origin and differentiation in the repair of full-thickness defects of articular cartilage. J Bone Joint Surg Am 1993; 75(4):532–53.

16. Lee KB, Bai LB, Yoon TR, et al. Second-look arthroscopic findings and clinical outcomes after microfracture for osteochondral lesions of the talus. Am J Sports Med 2009;37(Suppl 1):63s–70s.

17. Becher C, Driessen A, Hess T, et al. Microfracture for chondral defects of the talus: maintenance of early results at midterm follow-up. Knee Surg Sports Traumatol Arthrosc 2010;18(5):656–63.

18. Madry H, van Dijk CN, Mueller-Gerbl M. The basic science of the subchondral bone. Knee Surg Sports Traumatol Arthrosc 2010;18(4):419–33.

19. Chen H, Sun J, Hoemann CD, et al. Drilling and microfracture lead to different bone structure and necrosis during bone-marrow stimulation for cartilage repair. J Orthopaedic Res 2009;27(11):1432–8.

20. Orth P, Goebel L, Wolfram U, et al. Effect of subchondral drilling on the microarchitecture of subchondral bone: analysis in a large animal model at 6 months. Am J Sports Med 2012;40(4):828–36.

21. Seow D, Yasui Y, Hutchinson ID, et al. The subchondral bone is affected by bone marrow stimulation: a systematic review of preclinical animal studies. Cartilage 2019;10(1):70–81.

22. Brittberg M, Lindahl A, Nilsson A, et al. Treatment of deep cartilage defects in the knee with autologous chondrocyte transplantation. N Engl J Med 1994;331(14):889–95.

23. Kwak SK, Kern BS, Ferkel RD, et al. Autologous chondrocyte implantation of the ankle: 2- to 10-year results. Am J Sports Med 2014;42(9):2156–64.

24. Giannini S, Buda R, Ruffilli A, et al. Arthroscopic autologous chondrocyte implantation in the ankle joint. Knee Surg Sports Traumatol Arthrosc 2014; 22(6):1311–9.

25. Lenz CG, Tan S, Carey AL, et al. Matrix-induced autologous chondrocyte implantation (MACI) grafting for osteochondral lesions of the talus. Foot Ankle Int 2020;41(9):1099–105.

26. Giza E, Sullivan M, Ocel D, et al. Matrix-induced autologous chondrocyte implantation of talus articular defects. Foot Ankle Int 2010;31(9):747–53.

27. Lee YH, Suzer F, Thermann H. Autologous matrix-induced chondrogenesis in the knee: a review. Cartilage 2014;5(3):145–53.

28. Weigelt L, Hartmann R, Pfirrmann C, et al. Autologous matrix-induced chondrogenesis for osteochondral lesions of the talus: a clinical and radiological 2- to 8-year follow-up study. Am J Sports Med 2019;47(7):1679–86.

29. Giannini S, Buda R, Battaglia M, et al. One-step repair in talar osteochondral lesions: 4-year clinical results and t2-mapping capability in outcome prediction. Am J Sports Med 2013;41(3):511–8.

30. Giannini S, Buda R, Cavallo M, et al. Cartilage repair evolution in post-traumatic osteochondral lesions of the talus: from open field autologous chondrocyte to bone-marrow-derived cells transplantation. Injury 2010;41(11):1196–203.

31. Riff AJ, Davey A, Cole BJ. Emerging technologies in cartilage restoration. In: Yanke AB, Cole BJ, editors. Joint preservation of the knee: a clinical casebook. Cham (Switzerland): Springer International Publishing; 2019. p. 295–319.

32. Fortier LA, Chapman HS, Pownder SL, et al. BioCartilage improves cartilage repair compared with microfracture alone in an equine model of full-thickness cartilage loss. Am J Sports Med 2016; 44(9):2366–74.

33. Shimozono Y, Williamson ERC, Mercer NP, et al. Use of extracellular matrix cartilage allograft may improve infill of the defects in bone marrow stimulation for osteochondral lesions of the talus. Arthroscopy 2021;37(7):2262–9.

34. Shimozono Y, Hurley ET, Nguyen JT, et al. Allograft compared with autograft in osteochondral transplantation for the treatment of osteochondral lesions of the talus. J Bone Joint Surg Am 2018; 100(21):1838–44.

35. Migliorini F, Maffulli N, Baroncini A, et al. Allograft versus autograft osteochondral transplant for chondral defects of the talus: systematic review and meta-analysis. Am J Sports Med 2022;50(12):3447–55.

36. Kennedy JG, Murawski CD. The treatment of osteochondral lesions of the talus with autologous osteochondral transplantation and bone marrow aspirate concentrate: surgical technique. Cartilage 2011;2(4):327–36.

37. Nguyen A, Ramasamy A, Walsh M, et al. Autologous osteochondral transplantation for large osteochondral lesions of the talus is a viable option in an athletic population. Am J Sports Med 2019; 47(14):3429–35.

38. Everts P, Onishi K, Jayaram P, et al. Platelet-rich plasma: new performance understandings and

therapeutic considerations in 2020. Int J Mol Sci 2020;21(20). https://doi.org/10.3390/ijms21207794.

39. Danilkowicz RM, Grimm NL, Zhang GX, et al. Impact of early weightbearing after ankle arthroscopy and bone marrow stimulation for osteochondral lesions of the talus. Orthop J Sports Med 2021;9(9). 23259671211029883.

40. Görmeli G, Karakaplan M, Görmeli CA, et al. Clinical effects of platelet-rich plasma and hyaluronic acid as an additional therapy for talar osteochondral lesions treated with microfracture surgery: a prospective randomized clinical trial. Foot Ankle Int 2015;36(8):891–900.

41. Guney A, Akar M, Karaman I, et al. Clinical outcomes of platelet rich plasma (PRP) as an adjunct to microfracture surgery in osteochondral lesions of the talus. Knee Surg Sports Traumatol Arthrosc 2015;23(8):2384–9.

42. Seow D, Ubillus HA, Azam MT, et al. Limited evidence of adjuvant biologics with bone marrow stimulation for the treatment of osteochondral lesion of the talus: a systematic review. Knee Surg Sports Traumatol Arthrosc 2022. https://doi.org/10.1007/s00167-022-07130-z.

43. Boakye LA, Ross KA, Pinski JM, et al. Platelet-rich plasma increases transforming growth factor-beta1 expression at graft-host interface following autologous osteochondral transplantation in a rabbit model. World J Orthop 2015;6(11):961–9.

44. Smyth NA, Haleem AM, Murawski CD, et al. The effect of platelet-rich plasma on autologous osteochondral transplantation: an in vivo rabbit model. J Bone Joint Surg Am 2013;95(24):2185–93.

45. Russell RP, Apostolakos J, Hirose T, et al. Variability of platelet-rich plasma preparations. Sports Med Arthrosc Rev 2013;21(4):186–90.

46. Caplan AI. Mesenchymal stem cells. J Orthop Res 1991;9(5):641–50.

47. Fortier LA, Strauss EJ, Shepard DO, et al. Biological effects of bone marrow concentrate in knee pathologies. J Knee Surg 2019;32(1):2–8.

48. Barry F, Boynton RE, Liu B, et al. Chondrogenic differentiation of mesenchymal stem cells from bone marrow: differentiation-dependent gene expression of matrix components. Exp Cell Res 2001;268(2):189–200.

49. Fortier LA, Potter HG, Rickey EJ, et al. Concentrated bone marrow aspirate improves full-thickness cartilage repair compared with microfracture in the equine model. J Bone Joint Surg Am 2010;92(10):1927–37.

50. Wilke MM, Nydam DV, Nixon AJ. Enhanced early chondrogenesis in articular defects following arthroscopic mesenchymal stem cell implantation in an equine model. J Orthop Res 2007;25(7):913–25.

51. Murphy EP, McGoldrick NP, Curtin M, et al. A prospective evaluation of bone marrow aspirate concentrate and microfracture in the treatment of osteochondral lesions of the talus. Foot Ankle Surg 2019;25(4):441–8.

52. Mercer NP, Samsonov AP, Dankert JF, et al. Outcomes of autologous osteochondral transplantation with and without extracellular matrix cartilage allograft augmentation for osteochondral lesions of the talus. Am J Sports Med 2022;50(1):162–9.

53. Shimozono Y, Yasui Y, Hurley ET, et al. Concentrated bone marrow aspirate may decrease postoperative cyst occurrence rate in autologous osteochondral transplantation for osteochondral lesions of the talus. Arthroscopy 2019;35(1):99–105.

54. Doral MN, Bilge O, Batmaz G, et al. Treatment of osteochondral lesions of the talus with microfracture technique and postoperative hyaluronan injection. Knee Surg Sports Traumatol Arthrosc 2012;20(7):1398–403.

55. Kaplan LD, Lu Y, Snitzer J, et al. The effect of early hyaluronic acid delivery on the development of an acute articular cartilage lesion in a sheep model. Am J Sports Med 2009;37(12):2323–7.

56. Bajuri MY, Sabri S, Mazli N, et al. Osteochondral injury of the talus treated with cell-free hyaluronic acid-based scaffold (Hyalofast®) - a reliable solution. Cureus 2021;13(9):e17928.

57. Tahta M, Akkaya M, Gursoy S, et al. Arthroscopic treatment of osteochondral lesions of the talus: Nanofracture versus hyaluronic acid-based cell-free scaffold with concentration of autologous bone marrow aspirate. J Orthop Surg (Hong Kong) 2017;25(2). 2309499017717870.

58. Yontar NS, Aslan L, Can A, et al. One step treatment of talus osteochondral lesions with microfracture and cell free hyaluronic acid based scaffold combination. Acta Orthop Traumatol Turc 2019;53(5):372–5.

59. Colasanti CA, Mercer NP, Garcia JV, et al. In-office needle arthroscopy for the treatment of anterior ankle impingement yields high patient satisfaction with high rates of return to work and sport. Arthroscopy 2022;38(4):1302–11.

Spine

Technological Advances in Spine Surgery
Navigation, Robotics, and Augmented Reality

Tarek Yamout, MD[a], Lindsay D. Orosz, MS, PA-C[b],
Christopher R. Good, MD[a], Ehsan Jazini, MD[a],
Brandon Allen, BA[b], Jeffrey L. Gum, MD[c],*

KEYWORDS

- Spine • Surgery • Navigation • Robotics • Computer-assisted navigation • Augmented reality
- Pedicle screw

KEY POINTS

- Accurate screw placement is critical to avoid vascular or neurologic complications during spine surgery, resulting in the development and transformation of screw guidance or assist technologies within the past 3 decades.
- Computer-assisted navigation, robotic-guided spine surgery, and augmented reality surgical navigation are currently available technologies that have seen greater incorporation in the operating room.
- Each of these technologies has its advantages and disadvantages, and implementation must be carefully executed with appropriate understanding of how the technology functions and its limitations.

INTRODUCTION

Accurate screw placement is critical to avoid vascular or neurologic complications during spine surgery and to maximize fixation for fusion and deformity correction. As such, screw guidance or assist technologies have undergone significant evolution within the past 3 decades to enhance accuracy, precision, and reliability during instrumentation. In the traditional open screw insertion technique, trajectories were determined by exposing both the screw entry point and anatomic landmarks. Several drawbacks are associated with an open approach, including the utilization of large incisions coupled with tissue trauma and the disruption of adjacent structures.[1] To overcome these challenges, image-based navigation techniques were developed to offer a more minimally invasive approach. Minimally invasive surgery (MIS) is associated with a reduction in blood loss, length of hospital stay, and narcotic use in the postoperative period.[2,3] The consequence of an MIS approach is that direct visualization of relevant anatomic structures is forfeited or reduced.[4] However, as technology has advanced, indirect visualization has improved via assist technology.

The first step in the evolution was 2-dimensional imaging (fluoroscopic guidance), which was used for percutaneous instrumentation and continues to be a popular technique. Landmarks that would have been visualized directly in an open approach can be indirectly visualized

---

[a] Virginia Spine Institute, 11800 Sunrise Valley Drive, Suite 800, Reston, VA 20191, USA; [b] National Spine Health Foundation, 11800 Sunrise Valley Drive, Suite 330, Reston, VA 20191, USA; [c] Norton Leatherman Spine Center, 210 East Gray Street Suite 900, Louisville, KY 40202, USA
* Corresponding author.
E-mail address: Jlgum001@gmail.com

Orthop Clin N Am 54 (2023) 237–246
https://doi.org/10.1016/j.ocl.2022.11.008
0030-5898/23/© 2022 Elsevier Inc. All rights reserved.

during fluoroscopy in the anterior-posterior and lateral planes. Advantages with this technology include its versatility across a variety of different procedures, low operating cost, and fast learning curve.[1] However, the main limitations with fluoroscopic guidance are a lack of 3-dimensional (3D) understanding and the significant radiation exposure to the patient and operating room (OR) staff, with exposure being reported in one study as double when compared with freehand screw placement.[5]

The development of faster computer processors and advanced imaging technology allowed for successful integration of real-time information with 3D anatomy, called computer-assisted navigation (CAN), which has become increasingly popular.[6] CAN has been shown to improve workflow in the OR and increase both safety and accuracy in minimally invasive instrumentation when compared with freehand or fluoroscopic-guided screw placement.[6–9] In addition, a significant benefit for using CAN is the reduction in radiation exposure for both the OR staff and patient.[10,11]

Robotic guidance (RG) expands upon CAN by incorporating a robotic arm that provides a trajectory for pedicle screw instrumentation. RG can be further divided into 2 groups: robotic arms controlled by navigation (RAN) and automated anatomy recognition-based RG, of which the latter does not depend on optical navigation. RG exhibits several potential advantages when compared with fluoroscopic guidance including an increased ability for surgical planning and decreased risk of surgical complication, revision surgery, and significantly less radiation exposure.[4,12] Fluoroscopic guidance was also found to be less accurate with pedicle screw placement when compared with automated anatomy recognition-based RG.[13]

Augmented reality (AR) surgical navigation is a relatively novel screw guidance technology that operates by superimposing relevant anatomic structures, possible screw trajectories, as well as ideal screw locations onto the surgical field. Images identifying important structures can be obtained from both preoperative and intraoperative scans. This image projection onto the surgical field enables the surgeon to maintain a line of sight with the patient while operating, allowing proper orientation in the limited field of view that is a known accompaniment to MIS.[1,14]

The purpose of this review is to provide an overview of the current technologies available within CAN, RG, and AR, including details about the different operating systems available, their effects on efficiency and safety, radiation exposure, OR workflow, overall cost, learning curve, and future trends in spine surgery assistive technology.

DISCUSSION
3D Image-Based Computer-Assisted Navigation
Platforms

Successful use of CAN with 3D imaging for placement of open lumbar pedicle screws was first described in the literature in 1995.[6] Since then, there has been a concurrent development of CAN from a multitude of companies for use in both open and MIS spine surgery. In general, CAN systems use an optic sensor to coordinate relevant spinal anatomy with surgical instruments, using reference markers from a fixed frame attached either to bony anatomy (spine/pelvis) or to the skin.[15]

The Airo Mobile Intraoperative computed tomography (CT)-based CAN platform (Brainlab, Feldkirchen, Germany) is one of the earlier navigation platforms used in spine surgery, gaining US Food and Drug Administration (FDA) approval in 2013. Workflow for this system is as follows: (1) once the patient is positioned, prepped, and draped, three reference points attached to instruments used in this system are calibrated with the camera before intraoperative scanning; (2) a 360° CT scanner is deployed; (3) the reference points are then coupled with an anatomic reference clamp that is attached to an exposed spinous process or to the iliac crest via pins in percutaneous cases; and (4) an image is generated that is automatically registered to the platform's software thereby resulting in a real-time 3D image. Of note, the reference clamps or pins cannot be moved after registration with the system's camera due to shift in the registration, which would then necessitate a repeat scan.[6]

The StealthStation S8 with O-arm (Medtronic, Minneapolis, MN, USA) and the ZiehmVision FD Vario 3-D with NaviPort integration (Ziehm Imaging, Orlando, FL, USA) are similar CAN operating systems, which were FDA approved in 2017 and 2020, respectively. Medtronic had released its first O-arm system in 2006, having undergone a series of evolutions since then. The former uses an O-arm with 360° of rotation that opens at 90° to better mobilize around the patient. The latter uses a C-arm that obtains images via 190° rotation around the patient before reformatting those images into a 3D anatomic map. Both technologies have a reference registration system similar to the Airo Mobile platform, and as a result face a similar limitation that any movement of reference clamps can lead to inaccurate registration; this would necessitate repeat scanning, which increases the length of surgery and radiation exposure.[6]

The NAV3i platform with SpineMask Tracker and SpineMap Software (Stryker, Kalamazoo, MI, USA) was FDA approved in 2014 and differs from the aforementioned technologies because the SpineMask Tracker operates with a noninvasive form of referencing. This rectangular adhesive tracker is affixed to the patient's skin surrounding the area of interest, which avoids obstruction of the system's camera due to hand positioning or movement of reference points after calibration. Once the tracker is in place, registration occurs automatically using the SpineMap software algorithm to match the imaging to the patient's anatomy. The size of the operative field is limited by the predefined size parameters of the reference points, and excessive skin tension or deep retraction can result in inaccurate mapping, thereby constraining use of this device to MIS. If a surgeon elects to use this device for a large, open surgery then reference points must be placed at an area distal from the surgical wound that would be unaffected by retraction.[6] Stryker's Q Guidance system, FDA approved in June 2022, is its latest CAN release; however, there is no published literature about its clinical efficacy at this time. This system features a high-performance camera and redesigned software, and is the first navigation software to receive FDA clearance with pediatric patients as young as 13 years.

The 7D Surgical System (SeaSpine, Carlsbad, CA, USA) was FDA approved in 2021 and uses a relatively novel technology called machine vision navigation. Machine vision combines video cameras with computer systems to create an image. Workflow for this system is as follows: (1) once the patient is positioned, prepped, and draped, the device is placed next to the operating table with its head consisting of a surgical lamp, cameras, and light projector positioned above the surgical field; (2) the light projector is coupled with the 2 stereoscopic cameras to create a 3D image of exposed anatomy; and (3) the image is coregistered with a preoperatively or intraoperatively obtained CT or fluoroscopic image in seconds. If the reference array is moved, reregistration can be repeated without the need for repeat CT or fluoroscopic imaging, which allows for less radiation exposure when compared with other CAN devices. A limitation of this device is that the system head requires visualization of spinal surface anatomy for registration, which negates the ability to perform percutaneous instrumentation.[16]

Benefits and limitations

Several studies have investigated radiation exposure in spine surgery with CAN compared with fluoroscopic guidance.[11,17–21] With fluoroscopic guidance, there is significant radiation exposure for the surgeon and OR staff. Spine surgeons are susceptible to radiation exposure, facing 50 times the amount of radiation over the course of their career compared with other orthopedic surgeons.[22] Use of CAN in spine surgery has been demonstrated to reduce radiation exposure to OR staff and surgeons by at least a factor of 10.[20,21] Gebhard and colleagues,[19] in their 2006 study, reported that surgeons who used CAN for thoracolumbar instrumentation were exposed to a median radiation dose of 432 mSv as opposed to a dose of 1091 mSv using fluoroscopy with an average time of 40 seconds. A study by Kim and colleagues[10] demonstrated that CAN reduces fluoroscopy time by up to 90 seconds per case, significantly reducing exposure for the surgeon, who in some cases can leave the room while a scan is being conducted, thereby avoiding radiation. It is important to note that there is a variation in the amount of fluoroscopy used among spine surgeons, and radiation doses in some cases may be comparable to that for a singular intraoperative CT.[21,23]

There have been several studies conducted to evaluate the accuracy of CAN.[24–41] In a study by Amiot and colleagues,[39] the error rate with pedicle screw placement was compared between CAN and freehand techniques. Screws placed from T5 to S1 with freehand technique had a malposition rate of 15.3% for 544 screws as opposed to 5.4% for 294 screws inserted via CAN.[39] Yu and colleagues[32] similarly demonstrated that screws placed with CAN breached pedicles by more than 2 mm 4.6% of the time as opposed to a 16% malposition rate when using freehand technique. Luther and colleagues[37] compared pedicle breach between CAN (12%) and lateral fluoroscopy (18%). Towner and colleagues[40] compared 271 cases using CAN with 419 cases using fluoroscopy or freehand technique. The investigators found that only 1.1% of CAN cases required revision due to improperly positioned hardware as opposed to 2.4% of fluoroscopy or freehand cases, although these differences were not statistically significant.[40] In a study by Baky and colleagues,[41] they comparably found that 1% of screws placed using CAN had a 4-mm breach as opposed to 3.3%

of those placed via fluoroscopy ($P = .27$). In addition, 3.6% of fluoroscopy cases required a return to the OR, whereas 0% of cases using CAN returned to the OR ($P = .02$).[41] These studies demonstrate that computer-assisted navigated screw placement is associated with increased accuracy, and less complications, when compared with more traditional methods.

Despite its reported advantages regarding accuracy, safety, and radiation exposure, CAN also has some limitations. One potential drawback is the steep learning curve. Sclafani and colleagues[42] reported that novice surgeons learning how to perform percutaneous screw insertion using CAN with an O-arm had slower insertion times without loss of accuracy compared with those using traditional fluoroscopy who had faster insertion times but experienced reduced accuracy. Of note, accuracy did not suffer because operational speed improved throughout the training process with CAN.[42]

CAN has high upfront equipment costs, with platforms costing anywhere from $175,000 to $700,000 USD, with implementation costs and contracting contributing to variability in pricing.[43] Despite this high upfront financial investment, studies have demonstrated that there is a reduced rate of revision surgery when CAN is used, which in turn results in significant cost savings.[44–46] Drazin and colleagues[46] reported that the cost of a revision spine surgery ranges from $17,650 to $39,643 USD following a systematic cost analysis. This finding illustrates that the high upfront investment can be mitigated by avoiding revision spine surgery, which can result in significant savings. Similarly, Zausinger and colleagues[45] reported an average savings of $27,813.18 USD when revision surgeries are avoided in a 2-year retrospective analysis.

Robotic-Guided Spine Surgery
Platforms
Pedicle screw instrumentation using RG arose in the late 1990s, with the first clinical reports in the mid-2000s, partially out of a concern about screw malposition rates and radiation exposure with other MIS instrumentation techniques.[15,47,48] All current FDA-approved and commonly used spine robotic-assist systems operate under the principle of shared control, meaning that the robot functions in tandem with the surgeon who is the primary controller in the procedure.[47,48] The theory behind shared control systems is that they are able to reduce human error via increased accuracy, decreased fatigue, motion scaling, and tremor suppression via mechanical aid.[49]

The Mazor family of robotic systems (SpineAssist [Mazor Robotics Ltd, Caesarea, Israel], Mazor Renaissance, Mazor X, and Mazor X Stealth Edition [MXSE; Medtronic Minneapolis, MN, USA]) all have evolved using a core technology that includes automated anatomy recognition-based RG in which the robotic system is rigidly attached to the patient using some type of "bony mount." The Mazor SpineAssist, FDA approved in 2004, was the first spine surgery robot approved in the United States, and the second-generation Mazor Renaissance was released in 2011. This device offered improvements over the prior iteration, including upgraded image recognition algorithms and prevention of skidding of the guiding cannula along sloped anatomy.[48] The third-generation Mazor X, FDA approved in 2016, offered significant advantages over prior models, most importantly increased arm reach and strength. The robotic arm includes a linear optic camera that enables the robot to make a real-time volumetric assessment of the surgical field to increase accuracy and avoid collision intraoperatively.[48] Another benefit offered by the Mazor X is its serial, as opposed to parallel, robotic arm, which allows for a greater range of motion as well as a reduction in the need for additional surgical tools.[4,15,47,48,50] The Mazor X Align application allows for better preoperative planning and can simulate the impact of corrective changes on alignment. The ROSA Spine Robot (Zimmer Biomet Wilson, IN, USA), FDA approved in 2016, operates similarly to the Mazor X with the exception that it consists of 2 separate stands for its robotic arm and navigation camera. The MXSE, FDA approved in 2018 and first used in January 2019, integrates the Mazor X robotic system with Medtronic's Stealth navigation. With the parallel integration of navigated instruments, real-time feedback on instrument position along with 3D visualization of preoperatively planned screw trajectories is now possible. In addition, the MXSE interfaces with the patient directly. The robot is mounted to both the patient and the bed independent of optical tracking arrays that would otherwise be susceptible to movement or camera blockage, thereby enabling the robot to adjust to changes in the patient's position while maintaining its target trajectory.[12,47,50]

With the concurrent benefits of CAN, modern spine RAN platforms are now integrated with CAN systems.[15,47,50] The Excelsius GPS (Globus Medical Inc, Audubon, PA, USA), FDA approved in 2017, was one of the first integrated platforms released in the United States that allowed for real-time instrument tracking, intraoperative imaging, compensation for patient movement, and guidance of pedicle screw placement without the use of K-wires. The optical camera used for registration and tracking uses an intraoperative CT; however, the robot is capable of registration using a preoperative CT scan as well.[47,48] Similar to the MXSE, the ROSA platform acquired an FDA-approved upgrade in 2019 that includes a fully integrated CAN.[47]

Benefits and limitations

It is important to note that there are significant differences between robotic guidance systems in terms of hardware, but more importantly as it relates to the software, anatomy recognition, and registration. As such, research related to one type of robotic system cannot be applied or assumed to carry over to other systems.

eMany studies have reported a decrease in radiation exposure with RG.[4,47,48,51–54] In an RCT comparing fluoroscopic-guided pedicle screw placement and RAN, Roser and colleagues[54] demonstrated that the intraoperative radiation exposure was decreased by half in the RAN cohort. In systematic reviews by Peng and colleagues[52] and Fatima and colleagues,[51] intraoperative radiation exposure was significantly reduced in the RAN cohort compared with the freehand cohort by 12.4 and 3.7 seconds, respectively. In the MIS ReFRESH study by Good and colleagues,[4] RG with the Renaissance system reduced fluoroscopy time per screw by 80% (up to 1 minute per case) when compared with fluoroscopic guidance, and the total average intraoperative radiation exposure per RG case was less than half of the exposure per fluoroscopic case. In their multicenter cohort study, Lee and colleagues[50] compared navigated versus nonnavigated Mazor cohorts and found that the former had significantly shorter fluoroscopy time and mean fluoroscopy time per screw. All these findings demonstrate the potential RG has for reduced intraoperative radiation exposure compared with more conventional techniques.

There has been extensive research on the overall safety profile of bone-mounted RG.[4,48,50,53,55–58] In a multicenter database assessment, Lee and colleagues[57] found that patients who underwent lumbar fusion with RG had a low (4.4%) 1-year reoperation rate. Robot-related factors such as robot time per screw, open or percutaneous approach, and the specific robotic system used were not found to be independent factors influencing the 1-year reoperation rate. However, robot-related complications such as intraoperative exchange of screw (0.9%),

robot abandonment (2.5%), and return to the OR for screw exchange (1.3%) were found to increase the risk for greater blood loss and longer length of stay.[57] Good and colleagues[4] demonstrated that within a 1-year follow-up period the risk of complications was 5.8 times lower in the bone-mounted RG cohort compared with the fluoroscopic guidance cohort. The risk of a revision surgery was also 11.0 times lower for the RG cohort.[4] Yu and colleagues[58] demonstrated that patients undergoing a 1- to 3-level robotic-assisted posterior lumbar fusion did not have an increased 90-day complication rate compared with nonrobotic-assisted groups. Of note, there was an improvement in length of stay in the robotic-assisted group (2.5 vs 3.17 days, $P = .018$).[58] The literature supports the safety profile of RG.

Several studies have also determined screw placement accuracy with RG.[48,50,55,56] D'Souza and colleagues[48] noted that RG was more accurate and resulted in higher fusion rates than fluoroscopy-assisted procedures with a 95.3% and 86.9% fusion rate ($P = .038$), respectively. In a separate study evaluating S2AI screw placement via RG, Good and colleagues[55] found that RG is a reliable technique for accurate screw placement; 100% of screws graded for accuracy using postoperative CT scans were found to have 0 mm of breach. There was no significant difference in accuracy between RG integrated with CAN and nonnavigated RG cohorts when these were compared.[50] In their 5-year multi-center study on trends in RG, Lee and colleagues[56] found that screw accuracy, operative workflow, radiation exposure, rates of robot abandonment, and complication rates all improved at 4 institutions among 7 different surgeons between 2015 and 2019. Overall, the literature seems to support the accuracy of RG.

A potential limitation in the implementation of RG for institutions is the high upfront capital cost. Platforms may range in price anywhere from $550,000 to $1,100,000 USD. The price variability is attributed to the specific platform purchased as well as contracting. In addition, disposables and adjunct implants may contribute upward of $1500 USD in additional charges per case.[59] There is a paucity of multicenter cost-effectiveness studies; however, the MIS ReFRESH study did examine parameters that reflect cost savings such as radiation exposure, overall time in the operative room, and revision rates. RG was found to have a reduced risk for surgical complications and revision rates as well as significantly reduced fluoroscopy exposure.[4] In a single-center study, Gum and colleagues[60] examined cost-saving parameters between patients undergoing traditional open thoracolumbar interbody fusion (tTLIF), midline interbody fusion (MIDLIF), and their newly developed robotic-assisted MIDLIF (RA-MIDLIF) technique and found that patients undergoing RA-MIDLIF had a shorter average length of stay (1.53 days) compared with MIDLIF (2.71 days) and tTLIF (3.58 days). Additionally, MIDLIF and RA-MIDLIF had lower estimated blood loss and less OR time when compared with tTLIF.[60] Another single-center study examining cost-effectiveness at an academic center demonstrated that utilization of RG saved $608,546 USD in 1 year.[61] Despite its high upfront cost, RG has the potential to be cost effective upon implementation based on the available literature.

Several studies have investigated the learning curve associated with implementing RG.[62–65] Procedural efficiency and accuracy were not found to be markedly different between experienced and novice RG users; however, performance improved as more experience was attained.[62,63,65] Siddiqui and colleagues[64] investigated the learning curve with a full navigation-enabled platform, the Excelsius GPS, and found that there was no noticeable difference in performance between experienced surgeons and trainees when using RAN with full navigation thereby suggesting that efficiency is easily transferable via observation. Further investigations into learning curve with RG are warranted, yet these early findings on the latest enabling technologies are promising.

Augmented Reality
Platforms

AR navigation in spine surgery is the most novel of the current approaches to the guidance of pedicle screw placement. Worldwide, there are 2 subtypes of AR technology that are used: AR-based head-mounted displays (AR-HMD) and AR surgical navigation systems with an image display on a computer, tablet PC, or video projector (ARSN).[66] At present, there are only 2 AR-HMD devices approved in the United States.

The xvision-Spine System (Augmedics, Ltd, Chicago, IL, USA), FDA approved in 2019, is the first AR-HMD approved in the United States. The device operates by superimposing relevant anatomic structures, possible screw trajectories, as well as ideal screw locations onto the surgical field.[14] The VisAR system (Novarad, Provo, UT, USA) is the second AR-HMD available for use in the United States since gaining FDA approval in 2022. This software works with Microsoft's HoloLens 2 (Microsoft Corporation, Redmond,

WA, USA), transforming preoperative CT or fluoroscopic images into 3D virtual images, which are superimposed onto the patient. Of note, the device can respond to the surgeon's voice commands thereby allowing them to maintain focus on the procedure.[67]

Benefits and limitations

AR is advantageous with regard to reducing radiation exposure. Both currently available technologies only require a single preoperative or intraoperative CT scan for an entire procedure to be performed.[66] Carl and colleagues[68] implemented a low-dose protocol for intraoperative CT scanning, which they integrated with preoperative multimodal imaging for registration of the ARSN device. The investigators found that radiation exposure was reduced by about 70% when using this protocol.[68] This study was an attempt to establish a workflow for AR-assisted surgery with reduced radiation exposure. It is important to note that the literature on the implementation of AR in spine surgery and its effects on radiation exposure is limited, therefore more research needs to be conducted on the topic.

AR-assisted spine surgery has been demonstrated to be accurate and safe.[14,69,70] Elmi-Terander and colleagues[69] demonstrated that pedicle screw placement in minimally invasive thoracolumbar surgery using ARSN can be accurate without the use of intraoperative fluoroscopy or x-ray. The investigators had an 89% accuracy rate, with only 2 screws breaching 2 to 4 mm through the pedicle out of a total of 18.[69] In a follow-up matched-control study, they compared ARSN to traditional free-hand technique. The number of clinically accurate screws was higher in the ARSN cohort than the free-hand cohort, with a 93.9% and 89.6% rate, respectively ($P < .05$). In addition, only 36.6% of the ARSN cohort had a cortical breach compared with 69.4% for the free-hand cohort ($P < .001$).[70] Jazini and colleagues, in their prospective cohort study, examined accuracy and safety using AR-HMD. Screws were assessed for accuracy using the Gertzbein-Robbins (G-R) scale, and of the 208 screws, 97.1% were deemed to have a clinically accurate G-R grade of A or B (91.8% Grade A and 5.3% Grade B). Additionally, there were no early postoperative complications or revisions during the 2-week follow-up period.[14] Similarly, Liu and colleagues[71] found a screw accuracy rate of 98% based on grade A or B G-R scores following placement of 205 pedicle screws in their study using AR-HMD. Early safety and accuracy of AR-assisted spine surgery is promising; long-term research is needed to further evaluate safety parameters with this technology.

Current, FDA approved, AR-HMD can range from $60,000 to $300,000 USD with variation attributed to the platform and contracting.[72] The capital required to purchase and implement these technologies may be prohibitive for some hospital systems but is notably less than other enabling technologies. Multicenter studies regarding cost-effectiveness upon implementation of AR in spine surgery should be conducted in the future.

SUMMARY

Spine surgery has experienced significant and rapid evolution over the past 3 decades with regard to assistive technology. With the advent of multiple generations of new technologies, surgeons now have a diverse array of choices when it comes to pedicle screw placement technologies. Each of the technologies mentioned in this article has its advantages and disadvantages, and implementation must be carefully executed with appropriate understanding of how the technology functions and its limitations. Considerations for patient safety and optimal outcomes must be paramount.

In a technology-driven world, future advancements within spine surgery are inevitable. We have already seen the CAN/RAN integration with an inevitable CAN/RAN/AR integration soon. Will the function of the robotic arms become more independent and go beyond trajectory guidance? Will software upgrades use artificial intelligence to determine ideal alignment, deformity correction, and implant size/shape and then perform 3D printing? This is indeed an exciting era with countless possibilities.

CLINICS CARE POINTS

- Accurate screw placement is critical to avoid vascular or neurologic complications during spine surgery, resulting in the development and transformation of screw guidance or assist technologies within the past 3 decades.
- Computer-assisted navigation, robotic-guided spine surgery, and AR surgical navigation are currently available technologies that have seen greater incorporation in the OR.
- Each of these technologies has its advantages and disadvantages, and implementation must be carefully executed with appropriate understanding of how the technology functions and its limitations.

DISCLOSURE

Dr C.R. Good reports personal fees from Stryker/K2M, personal fees from Medtronic, personal fees from Augmedics, and personal fees from NSite. Dr E. Jazini has served as a consultant for Stryker, Medtronic, and Innovasis. The authors have nothing else to disclose. Consultant – Acuity, Depuy, Medtronic, NuVasive, Stryker, FYR Medical, Expanding Innovations Royalties – Acuity, Medtronic, NuVasiveHonorarium – Pacira Pharmaceuticals, Baxter, Broadwater, NASS, MiMedx Advisory Board – Medtronic, National Spine Health Foundation, FYR Medical Journal Reviewer – The Spine Journal, Spine Deformity, Global Spine JournalResearch Support – Alan L. & Jacqueline B. Stuart Spine Center, Biom'Up, Cerapedics, Inc., Empirical Spine, Inc. Medtronic, National Spine Health Foundation, Pfizer, Scoliosis Research Society, Stryker, Texas Scottish Rites Hospital Speaking - KyANANorton Healthcare – Research Funding Stock: Cingulate Therapeutics, FYR MedicalShared Patents – Medtronic-Grants – Fischer Owen Fund – Travel Funds.

REFERENCES

1. Goldberg JL, Kirnaz S, Carnevale JA, et al. History of navigation guided spine surgery. In: Kim J, Hartl R, Wang M, et al, editors. Technical advances in minimally invasive spine surgery, vol. 1, 1st edition. Singapore: Springer Nature; 2022. p. 3–10.
2. Nerland US, Jakola AS, Solheim O, et al. Minimally invasive decompression versus open laminectomy for central stenosis of the lumbar spine: pragmatic comparative effectiveness study. BMJ 2015; 350(apr01 1):h1603.
3. Imada A, Huynh TR, Drazin D. Minimally invasive versus open laminectomy/discectomy, transforaminal lumbar, and posterior lumbar interbody fusions: a systematic review. Cureus 2017;9(7). https://doi.org/10.7759/cureus.1488.
4. Good CR, Orosz L, Schroerlucke SR, et al. Complications and revision rates in minimally invasive robotic-guided versus fluoroscopic-guided spinal fusions: the mis refresh prospective comparative study. Spine (Phila Pa 1976) 2021; 46(23):1661–8.
5. Tian NF, Wu YS, Zhang XL, et al. Minimally invasive versus open transforaminal lumbar interbody fusion: a meta-analysis based on the current evidence. Eur Spine J 2013;22(8):1741–9.
6. Rawicki N, Dowdell JE, Sandhu HS. Current state of navigation in spine surgery. Ann Transl Med 2021; 9(1). https://doi.org/10.21037/atm-20-1335.
7. Hussain I, Navarro-Ramirez R, Lang G, et al. 3D Navigation-guided resection of giant ventral cervical intradural schwannoma with 360-degree stabilization. Clin Spine Surg 2018;31(5):E257–65.

8. Navarro-Ramirez R, Lang G, Lian X, et al. Total navigation in spine surgery; a concise guide to eliminate fluoroscopy using a portable intraoperative computed tomography 3-dimensional navigation system. World Neurosurg 2017;100: 325–35.

9. Janssen I, Lang G, Navarro-Ramirez R, et al. Can fan-beam interactive computed tomography accurately predict indirect decompression in minimally invasive spine surgery fusion procedures? World Neurosurg 2017;107:322–33.

10. Kim CW, Lee YP, Taylor W, et al. Use of navigation-assisted fluoroscopy to decrease radiation exposure during minimally invasive spine surgery. Spine J 2008;8(4):584–90.

11. Kraus MD, Krischak G, Keppler P, et al. Can computer-assisted surgery reduce the effective dose for spinal fusion and sacroiliac screw insertion? Clin Orthopaedics Relat Res 2010;468(9): 2419–29.

12. Buza JA, Good CR, Lehman RA, et al. Robotic-assisted cortical bone trajectory (CBT) screws using the Mazor X Stealth Edition (MXSE) system: workflow and technical tips for safe and efficient use. J Robotic Surg 2021;15(1):13–23.

13. Fan Y, Du J, Zhang J, et al. Comparison of accuracy of pedicle screw insertion among 4 guided technologies in spine surgery. Med Sci Monitor 2017;23: 5960–8.

14. Bhatt FR, Orosz LD, Tewari A, et al. Augmented reality-assisted spine surgery: an early experience demonstrating safety and accuracy with 218 screws. Glob Spine J 2022;0(0):1–6.

15. Garg S, Kleck CJ, Gum JL, et al. Navigation options for spinal surgeons: state of the art 2021. Instr Course Lect 2022;71:399–411.

16. Kalfas IH. Machine vision navigation in spine surgery. Front Surg 2021;8. https://doi.org/10.3389/fsurg.2021.640554.

17. Gebhard F, Kraus M, Schneider E, et al. Radiation dosage in orthopedics – a comparison of computer-assisted procedures. Unfallchirurg 2003; 106(6):492–7.

18. Gebhard F, Weidner A, Liener UC, et al. Navigation at the spine. Injury 2004;35(1):35–45.

19. Gebhard FT, Kraus MD, Schneider E, et al. Does Computer-Assisted Spine Surgery Reduce Intraoperative Radiation Doses? Spine (Phila Pa 1976) 2006;31(17):2024–7.

20. Smith H, Welsch M, Ugurlu H, et al. Comparison of radiation exposure in lumbar pedicle screw placement with fluoroscopy vs computer-assisted image guidance with intraoperative three-dimensional imaging. J Spinal Cord Med 2008;31(5):532–7.

21. Nelson EM, Monazzam SM, Kim KD, et al. Intraoperative fluoroscopy, portable X-ray, and CT: patient and operating room personnel radiation exposure in spinal surgery. Spine J 2014;14(12): 2985–91.

22. Theocharopoulos N, Perisinakis K, Damilakis J, et al. Occupational Exposure from Common Fluoroscopic Projections Used in Orthopaedic Surgery. J Bone Joint Surg 2003;85(9):1698–703.

23. Jones DPG, Robertson PA, Lunt B, et al. Radiation exposure during fluoroscopically assisted pedicle screw insertion in the lumbar spine. Spine (Phila Pa 1976) 2000;25(12):1538–41.

24. Nakashima H, Sato K, Ando T, et al. Comparison of the percutaneous screw placement precision of isocentric C-arm 3-dimensional fluoroscopy-navigated pedicle screw implantation and conventional fluoroscopy method with minimally invasive surgery. J Spinal Disord Tech 2009; 22(7):468–72.

25. Merloz P, Troccaz J, Vouaillat H, et al. Fluoroscopy-based navigation system in spine surgery. Proc Inst Mech Eng H 2007;221(7):813–20.

26. Lee GYF, Massicotte EM, Raja Rampersaud Y. Clinical accuracy of cervicothoracic pedicle screw placement. J Spinal Disord Tech 2007;20(1):25–32.

27. Laine T, Lund T, Ylikoski M, et al. Accuracy of pedicle screw insertion with and without computer assistance: a randomised controlled clinical study in 100 consecutive patients. Eur Spine J 2000;9(3): 235–40.

28. Kotani Y, Abumi K, Ito M, et al. Accuracy Analysis of Pedicle Screw Placement in Posterior Scoliosis Surgery. Spine (Phila Pa 1976) 2007;32(14):1543–50.

29. Kotani Y, Abumi K, Ito M, et al. Improved accuracy of computer-assisted cervical pedicle screw insertion. J Neurosurg 2003;99(3):257–63.

30. Ito H, Neo M, Yoshida M, et al. Efficacy of computer-assisted pedicle screw insertion for cervical instability in RA patients. Rheumatol Int 2007; 27(6):567–74.

31. Ishikawa Y, Kanemura T, Yoshida G, et al. Clinical accuracy of three-dimensional fluoroscopy-based computer-assisted cervical pedicle screw placement: a retrospective comparative study of conventional versus computer-assisted cervical pedicle screw placement. J Neurosurg 2010;13(5):606–11.

32. Yu X, Xu L, yan Bi L. [Spinal navigation with intraoperative 3D-imaging modality in lumbar pedicle screw fixation]. Zhonghua Yi Xue Za Zhi 2008; 88(27):1905–8.

33. Yson SC, Sembrano JN, Sanders PC, et al. Comparison of cranial facet joint violation rates between open and percutaneous pedicle screw placement using intraoperative 3-D CT (O-arm) computer navigation. Spine (Phila Pa 1976) 2013;38(4):E251–8.

34. Verma SK, Singh PK, Agrawal D, et al. O-arm with navigation versus C-arm: a review of screw placement over 3 years at a major trauma center. Br J Neurosurg 2016;30(6):658–61.

35. van de Kelft E, Costa F, van der Planken D, et al. A prospective multicenter registry on the accuracy of pedicle screw placement in the thoracic, lumbar, and sacral levels with the use of the o-arm imaging system and stealthstation navigation. Spine (Phila Pa 1976) 2012;37(25):E1580–7.

36. Shin MH, Ryu KS, Park CK. Accuracy and safety in pedicle screw placement in the thoracic and lumbar spines : comparison study between conventional c-arm fluoroscopy and navigation coupled with o-arm® guided methods. J Korean Neurosurg Soc 2012;52(3):204.

37. Luther N, Iorgulescu JB, Geannette C, et al. Comparison of navigated versus non-navigated pedicle screw placement in 260 patients and 1434 screws. J Spinal Disord Tech 2015;28(5):E298–303.

38. Larson AN, Santos ERG, Polly DW, et al. Pediatric pedicle screw placement using intraoperative computed tomography and 3-dimensional image-guided navigation. Spine (Phila Pa 1976) 2012;37(3):E188–94.

39. Amiot LP, Lang K, Putzier M, et al. Comparative results between conventional and computer-assisted pedicle screw installation in the thoracic, lumbar, and sacral spine. Spine (Phila Pa 1976) 2000;25(5):606–14.

40. Towner JE, Li YI, Singla A, et al. Retrospective review of revision surgery after image-guided instrumented spinal surgery compared with traditional instrumented spinal surgery. Clin Spine Surg 2020;33(7):E317–21.

41. Baky FJ, Milbrandt T, Echternacht S, et al. Intraoperative Computed Tomography–Guided Navigation for Pediatric Spine Patients Reduced Return to Operating Room for Screw Malposition Compared With Freehand/Fluoroscopic Techniques. Spine Deformity 2019;7(4):577–81.

42. Sclafani JA, Regev GJ, Webb J, et al. Use of a quantitative pedicle screw accuracy system to assess new technology: Initial studies on O-arm navigation and its effect on the learning curve of percutaneous pedicle screw insertion. SAS J 2011;5(3):57–62.

43. Malham GM, Wells-Quinn T. What should my hospital buy next?—Guidelines for the acquisition and application of imaging, navigation, and robotics for spine surgery. J Spine Surg 2019;5(1):155–65.

44. Overley SC, Cho SK, Mehta AI, et al. Navigation and robotics in spinal surgery: where are we now? Neurosurgery 2017;80(3S):S86–99.

45. Zausinger S, Scheder B, Uhl E, et al. Intraoperative computed tomography with integrated navigation system in spinal stabilizations. Spine (Phila Pa 1976) 2009;34(26):2919–26.

46. Drazin D, Al-Khouja L, Shweikeh F, et al. Economics of image guidance and navigation in spine surgery. Surg Neurol Int 2015;6(11):S323–6.

47. Huang M, Tetreault TA, Vaishnav A, et al. The current state of navigation in robotic spine surgery. Ann Transl Med 2021;9(1). https://doi.org/10.21037/atm-2020-ioi-07.

48. D'Souza M, Gendreau J, Feng A, et al. Robotic-assisted spine surgery: history, efficacy, cost, and future trends. Robotic Surg Res Rev 2019;6:9–23.

49. Nathoo N, Çavuşoğlu MC, Vogelbaum MA, et al. In touch with robotics: neurosurgery for the future. Neurosurgery 2005;56(3):421–33.

50. Lee NJ, Zuckerman SL, Buchanan IA, et al. Is there a difference between navigated and non-navigated robot cohorts in robot-assisted spine surgery? A multicenter, propensity-matched analysis of 2,800 screws and 372 patients. Spine J 2021;21(9):1504–12.

51. Fatima N, Massaad E, Hadzipasic M, et al. Safety and accuracy of robot-assisted placement of pedicle screws compared to conventional free-hand technique: a systematic review and meta-analysis. Spine J 2021;21(2):181–92.

52. Peng YN, Tsai LC, Hsu HC, et al. Accuracy of robot-assisted versus conventional freehand pedicle screw placement in spine surgery: a systematic review and meta-analysis of randomized controlled trials. Ann Translational Med 2020;8(13):824.

53. Lee NJ, Buchanan IA, Zuckermann SL, et al. What is the comparison in robot time per screw, radiation exposure, robot abandonment, screw accuracy, and clinical outcomes between percutaneous and open robot-assisted short lumbar fusion? a multicenter, propensity-matched analysis of 310 patients. Spine (Phila Pa 1976) 2022;47(1):42–8.

54. Roser F, Tatagiba M, Maier G. Spinal Robotics. Neurosurgery 2013;72(Supplement 1):A12–8.

55. Good CR, Orosz LD, Thomson AE, et al. Robotic-guidance allows for accurate S2AI screw placement without complications. J Robotic Surg 2021;0123456789:2–7.

56. Lee NJ, Leung E, Buchanan IA, et al. A multicenter study of the 5-year trends in robot-assisted spine surgery outcomes and complications. J Spine Surg 2022;8(1):9–20.

57. Lee NJ, Buchanan IA, Boddapati V, et al. Do robot-related complications influence 1 year reoperations and other clinical outcomes after robot-assisted lumbar arthrodesis? A multicenter assessment of 320 patients. J Orthopaedic Surg Res 2021;16(1). https://doi.org/10.1186/s13018-021-02452-z.

58. Yu CC, Carreon LY, Glassman SD, et al. Propensity-matched comparison of 90-day complications in robotic-assisted versus non-robotic assisted lumbar fusion. Spine (Phila Pa 1976) 2022;47(3):195–200.

59. Fiani B, Quadri SA, Farooqui M, et al. Impact of robot-assisted spine surgery on health care quality

and neurosurgical economics: A systemic review. Neurosurg Rev 2020;43(1):17–25.

60. Gum JL, Crawford CH, Djurasovic M, et al. Introducing navigation or robotics into TLIF techniques: are we optimizing our index episode of care or just spending more money? Spine J 2019;19(9):S61–2.

61. Menger RP, Savardekar AR, Farokhi F, et al. A cost-effectiveness analysis of the integration of robotic spine technology in spine surgery. Neurospine 2018;15(3):216–24.

62. Urakov TM, Chang KH, Burks SS, et al. Initial academic experience and learning curve with robotic spine instrumentation. Neurosurg Focus 2017; 42(5):E4.

63. Kam JKT, Gan C, Dimou S, et al. Learning curve for robot-assisted percutaneous pedicle screw placement in thoracolumbar surgery. Asian Spine J 2019;13(6):920–7.

64. Siddiqui MI, Wallace DJ, Salazar LM, et al. Robot-assisted pedicle screw placement: learning curve experience. World Neurosurg 2019;130: e417–22.

65. Hu X, Lieberman IH. What is the learning curve for robotic-assisted pedicle screw placement in spine surgery? Clin Orthopaedics Relat Res 2014;472(6): 1839–44.

66. Liu Y, Lee MG, Kim JS. Spine surgery assisted by augmented reality: where have we been? Yonsei Med J 2022;63(4):305–16.

67. Felix B, Kalatar SB, Moatz B, et al. Augmented reality spine surgery navigation. Spine (Phila Pa 1976) 2022;47(12):865–72.

68. Carl B, Bopp M, Saß B, et al. Implementation of augmented reality support in spine surgery. Eur Spine J 2019;28(7):1697–711.

69. Elmi-Terander A, Nachabe R, Skulason H, et al. Feasibility and accuracy of thoracolumbar minimally invasive pedicle screw placement with augmented reality navigation technology. Spine (Phila Pa 1976) 2018;43(14):1018–23.

70. Elmi-Terander A, Burström G, Nachabé R, et al. Augmented reality navigation with intraoperative 3D imaging vs fluoroscopy-assisted free-hand surgery for spine fixation surgery: a matched-control study comparing accuracy. Scientific Rep 2020;10(707):1–8.

71. Liu A, Jin Y, Cottrill E, et al. Clinical accuracy and initial experience with augmented reality-assisted pedicle screw placement: the first 205 screws. J Neurosurg Spine 2022;36(3):351–7.

72. Driver J, Groff MW. Editorial. Navigation in spine surgery: an innovation here to stay. J Neurosurg Spine 2022;36(3):347–9.

Printed and bound by CPI Group (UK) Ltd, Croydon, CR0 4YY

08/05/2025

01864715-0013